NATURE FIGHTS BACK

Nature Fights Back

The Mineral Activators - My Memoir

IRENE FISHER N.D. B.A. M.ED. (COUNSELLING & DEVELOPMENT)

A catalogue record for this book is available from the National Library of Australia

ISBN 978-0-6487123-0-5 (paperback)
ISBN 978-0-6487123-1-2 (ebook)

Cover Photo: Irene Fisher
Interior Layout: Automated composition (Pickawoowoo Publishing Group)
Cover Layout: Pickawoowoo Publishing Group
Print and Chanel Distribution: Lightning Source / Ingram

Disclaimer
It is noted that the references to mineral compounds in this text, where, as an example, potassium phosphate is referred to, this is a mineral compound which has been pharmaceutically produced at high quality, purity and a low dose product which over many years has proved safest for human consumption. This may not be the compound as used for gardening or similar. Minerals or herbal supplements are better prescribed by a qualified practising professional. Please note that the minerals are in what is known as the biochemical formula, with the cation or positive charge (i.e. potassium) always combining with the anion or negative charge (i.e. phosphate) for nature's specific purposes.

YOU CAN TRACE EVERY SICKNESS, EVERY DISEASE,
EVERY AILMENT ULTIMATELY TO A MINERAL DEFICIENCY.

- LINUS PAULING -

(PERMISSION NOT SOUGHT)

CONTENTS

INTRODUCTION

L ooking back over what I've written I realise that my allegiance to a single basic modality of restoring health probably developed from my childhood when at 12, I passionately wanted to know about life, the truth of life. More than anything I wanted to understand if there was God, an entity that we and all of life was dependant on and I was lucky enough to find in later life, that there is an intelligence in all of life which restores and regenerates when the elements of life, clean air and clean water are optimal.

I've seen what happens when we as a species of meddling monkey play God. I was about 12 when I began camping each year with friends, over the long weekend in June to Bunya Crossing. We did not take a tent. It did not rain in June, that is until, as we heard, our American friends let off a missile into the ionosphere off the Queensland coast in the early 1960s and the weather changed dramatically. At school we had been taught that we had a stable sub-tropical climate which meant it did not rain in winter. Humidity built up in early summer and the rain flooded down at the end of January when we went back to school and it rained for two solid weeks non stop. Our climate was steady and predictable. Weren't we clever to interfere with it!!!

Growing up in Queensland, in the 1950s most people were either Catholic or Protestant and both were quite polarised and hostile to one another. My father did not believe in religion, "the opium of the people," yet he was treated by everyone as a Christian. He was a quiet, gentle man who could grow plants out of season and people often came to see his flowers. Children and even very frightened animals trusted him and he could persuade any animal to come to him. He worked for the rights of the workers, unemployment benefits etc. and was on the local progress association.

I understood how he felt about the church. His father was in the British Army in India and Dad and his brothers were educated at a military school high in the Himalayas. It was harsh, very cold in winter. When Dad started school, he was a small boy. Each morning there was an inspection of beds and toiletries. If anything was missing one got the cuts. Dad, being new and small was vulnerable to things being pinched from his toiletry bag. The problem was solved when one of the Indian servants gave Dad a pet snake to live in his toiletry bag. Perhaps that was the beginning of a lifelong trust by animals in him. Every morning they went to church before a breakfast of porridge with molasses and weevils. One of his brothers ran away from the school, twice and twice he was returned and publicly flogged. Then they went to church after the floggings. The older brothers decided that church and Christianity were hypocritical.

We lived in a working class area, where, when the pay ran out, families sometimes lived on porridge until the next pay, no rubbishy food to harm their health then. My father did not drink or smoke so we lived a bit better. One of Dad's mates told me that my Dad was just like Jesus Christ, but with a fault - his tolerance of my volatile mother. I have seen my mother chase a cheeky larrikin down the street with lumps of wood for swearing at her. She and her mother believed in Womens Rights and my father happily helped with cooking and housework when this was unfashionable for men. My mother had a savage temper but was also an interesting mother who read to us each night, books like the KonTiki expedition. She was sought out by the neighbours in times of trouble. My father worked for the railways so we got a free pass on the trains each year and my mother organised wonderful camping holidays. I learned to swim on the Atherton Tableland where she grew up as a child. I was 7 and watched the Aborigine children swim to and from a little island in the pool at the foot of the Kuranda Falls and decided I could do that too. My Dad took me to a tree where there was a mother possum and her baby and each day we fed them bread. He found a paddock above the Malanda Falls where we were camped which was thick with vivid blue butterflies and we walked to Lakes Barrine and Eacham. At home where we lived, we were close to a wonderful creek and the bush. We children ran around barefooted and it was death adder country, but if we saw a snake, we stopped and waited. None of us were ever bitten.

Our house was full of books. I read a lot and got more and more interested in the question of the truth of our existence. I went to many churches of all denominations, but most of all loved the open-air Sunday School at the foot of our road, where we learned about Jesus and how he stood up for what he believed in. We were so fortunate to learn the stories of Christianity, of courage and conviction. Learning in all species is about knowledge being passed on. Now children so often grow up in a vacuum or a void, where the only truth is what our elites want taught at school which doesn't include religion, just as if we, who are created in nature have all the answers. Of course we require skills for earning a living, but we also need to learn from our history, so we can better understand our present life and certainly it is hypocritical to call ourselves a democracy, when our children do not learn the history of democracy, how other democracies work and /or the many kinds of battles fought for it. Knowing how to get on with each other is one thing, but equally important is to understand power struggles that are innate within us.

I was born during the second world war and was very fortunate to grow up in a simple world, where we had few possessions, but each others' company and a strong value system, that mostly stemmed from our various Christian religions. I was lucky to live on the edge of Brisbane, where we children lived such a rich, natural life. So I think that's why years later, the question of life and what was the truth became focussed from a conversation with Dr Maurice Blackmore. I took it seriously when he said that if one attended to the basics, the minerals, our electrolytes in the biochemical format of nature, and observed the symptoms discovered by previous generations of doctors, I would see the regeneration of health, not just of us, but of all creatures. The attainment of balance seems to be key to how Nature promotes life. So one can understand that superphosphate for Australian soils, with the anion of phosphate and the cations (potassium, magnesium, calcium, iron, sodium) needs to be a balanced formula. However in superphosphate, the amounts of cations combined with the anion of phosphate are in quite low amounts, which may well account for reported burning of the soil when superphosphate is applied. Certainly the phosphate promotes growth, but with insufficient of the cations for balance and may further promote lacks of the essential cations. In my memoir I tell a story of a man who showed excessive amounts of phosphorous in his blood test which fortunately responded to phosphate with cation minerals in what has been found to be a balanced formulation and the phosphorous level in his bloodstream became quickly normal and his health built up within weeks.

Over decades, I've finally understood that without these activators of life, there also becomes less energy and joy in life. I have never been able to accept the idea of "incurable." Within the miracle and complexity of life there is a great intelligence that promotes healing and balance. We, like all living things are ultimately subject to life's laws. Over recent years I've learned that the balance of life also becomes threatened by increasing levels of atmospheric carbon dioxide. My memoir tells the story of how I learned about the elements of life, how essential they are to all of life and how therefore we must get CO_2 back into balance or risk observing and experiencing all of life becoming more and more incapacitated with debilitating diseases including escalating chronic fatigue, learning difficulties and dementia. No minerals means no life.

Irene Fisher

Naturopath - N.D. B.A. M.Ed (Counselling & Development)

~ One ~

OVERSEAS, RETURN AND CHANGE OF DIRECTION.

In 1970 I had returned to Australia from the U.S.A. and England where I had lived and worked for nearly 10 years. I was 28 years old and it didn't occur to me that my experiences of life overseas would lead me to the beginnings of a new understanding about the importance of the most basic processes of health, that I'd not been exposed to before coming to live in Melbourne, where I had a favourite uncle and his family. (Brisbane, which was my home seemed too hot after Europe and I had also hated the heat of Texas. It also upset me that the housing estate now on either side of Kedron Brook which I had loved as a child seemed lifeless with only cicadas and other insects to hear. The birds and wildlife we children had loved were gone due to insecticides I was told and so was the pure rushing stream which now seemed dead and stagnant - not the home I remembered in my memory). In America I had read all of Adelle Davis's wonderful books about vitamins and had found her knowledge very useful. Now in Melbourne, I would learn about the minerals and see that the name "Blackmores" was at the forefront and seemed to be the foundation to a health revolution not seen in Europe or America.

In 1960 I'd sailed on the sleek white Fairsky to Europe. I was 18 years of age and was accompanied by my friend Joan to Italy for the Rome Olympics. It was the Melbourne Olympic Games that led to me leaving high school, working, saving and finishing my education at night school to go to the next Olympics. Australians then were a more reserved people, but loved sport as much then as today, the only thing they seemed to get emotional about. The hero of the games was a shy Russian called Vladimir Kutz and this was despite the Hungarian revolution only months earlier. At the closing ceremony, for the first time in Olympic history, the athletes broke ranks and came out with their arms around each other. Australia with its small population won the third highest tally in medals : U.S.A., USSR, then Australia. I was very idealistic and so became determined to go to the Games in Rome in 1960.

People did not fly then. We sailed down the Brisbane River up the Queensland coast in April, 1960. On our way we saw the terrible poverty in Singapore, the beauty of Mt Lavinia in Ceylon, then more terrible poverty in the Suez Canal. We docked at Aden and saw people living in houses made with newspaper, side by side with an American coca cola stand. Today in Yemen it's U.S. bombs from Saudi Arabia. At Cairo we rode camels to the Sphinx. We would not have guessed that within a few years, the Suez Canal with desert on both sides would be closed. We really were lucky to experience such a voyage.

We disembarked in Naples and hitch hiked all over Europe. At Hammerfest we saw the Midnight sun, stayed in Berlin a month and ate in East Berlin as the East German mark was one fifth the value of the West German mark (the wall going up a year later) was probably not surprising) and returned with our huge haversacks to Rome and a totally different Olympic games from Melbourne. At the closing ceremony only the flag bearers appeared - no athletes and no Olympic spirit. But we loved Italy, wonderful art galleries in even quite small towns and the great generosity of the Italian people.

We went to England. Joan went home to Brisbane and I stayed to study opera singing with another friend. We were secretaries in offices and waitresses in coffee shops, two jobs at a time. I got a job as secretary to the manager of the second largest gentlemens' clothing company in England and one day at lunchtime I stopped to admire jewellery in an arcade in Regent Street and at the back saw photos of dancers and showgirls in wonderful costumes. I suddenly wanted to escape from my life as a secretary and went downstairs and knocked. I bluffed my way into cabaret at Eves. I was lucky as they had suddenly become a girl short. Eves was a beautiful and well run club. I was very lucky as it was then the most exclusive club in London. We danced in two shows a night. I had to do ballet classes every day and was told by Helen Archer my boss, to smile so hopefully no one would look at my feet. I had a flat just off Baker Street in a wonderful old Robert Adams building, in Blandford Street, near osteopaths and complementary health shops in Baker Street. I loved walking home in the early hours after the last show, window-shopping and saying "hello" to the occasional policeman on the beat. Night life was safe then and I never developed fear until over a year later I went to America. My new American friends thought I was insulting America when I told them about walking home safely in the early hours of the morning in such a large city as London. They did not believe me. I worked for Pan Am, a wonderful airline but did not want to live in the U.S. long term and returned to Australia and then wondered what I would do next.

~ Two ~

NATUROPATHIC COLLEGE AND
MINERALS IN PRACTICE.

In Melbourne I met a shy young man at a party, who was in constant pain because of flaccid ligaments along his spine. He was told that nothing medically could be done. This meeting led to the great change of direction in my life and the subject of this book. Apart from my love of dancing, singing and theatre, I had also been a child who brought home sick animals, dogs that died of distemper. Looking back I realise how generous my family was as at teatime, after a death of an animal I could not eat and turned my brother off his food too. However, I could not accept that nothing could be done about this young man's constant back pain. The question stayed in my mind until one day I found an English health magazine in a health shop in Little Collins Street and saw an advertisement inside for Naturopaths. When I returned to work I looked up the pink pages (as the telephone directory was then) and to my surprise found listed naturopaths and a college.

The college was run by Alf Jacka, who originally was an electrical engineer. I became a student in 1970. The college was financed from Blackmores Laboratories in Sydney. I became an enthusiastic student. Herbalism was my favourite subject in the first year, which we studied along with anatomy and physiology. But it was in second year, just before the first class on the minerals that my introduction to another method of practice began.

On that first day I was sitting next to Hedley, an agronomist who had just returned from the U.K.

He said "Now we are getting somewhere."

"What do you mean, Hedley?" I asked.

He said "Have you never wondered why the English were known as the Bulldog species? No? It's because of their calcium rich soil and the Irish, why they have been known for their volatility? It relates to the lack of potassium in their soil?"

I was fascinated and later, in 1971 when I met Dr Maurice Blackmore at his home in Sydney and also visited Blackmore's laboratories, Dr Blackmore's words also fascinated me. "Why" I asked him, "Do you say the celloids (his name for his mineral compounds) are so important?'

He said "Girlie, these minerals are essential for structure and human metabolism and are often grossly lacking in Australia's ancient soils and where they are scarce in the soil, they are lacking in the food we eat. You will learn there are specific symptoms that show when these minerals are needed. Be guided by the symptoms. And don't be fooled by the Vitacelloids and other products the laboratories are now making. I founded the laboratories for the celloids."

I could not believe there was such a simple foundation to human health and if there was, why wasn't the medical profession on to it? At the same time, the only way to know was to try out the system and the only person who was using the celloids exclusively at that time was Les Fisher. Today I realise that Dr Maurice Blackmore is an as yet unsung Australian genius, a man of great courage who would not back down from what he learned. I was told that he had been reviled by the medical profession of his day.

Later I heard that Dr Maurice Blackmore founded the laboratories on the money won from broken down racehorses that he built up on his mineral compound powder. Years later I bought the last bag of this mineral compound for Sweet Pea, also a broken down racehorse we bought for my daughter in Tasmania.

Years later I met a biochemist from the Antarctic base in Tasmania, who came into Edwards Pharmacy in Kingston where I worked. He always made a beeline for the minerals. I asked him if he needed any help. "No. I know what my family and I need". I must have stared at him, because then he said "Our soils are grossly deficient. If you put an Australian animal under a spectrometer you can see how lacking in minerals the animals are. So I buy the minerals I think my family needs."

Only recently, I have learned something of the work of Linus Pauling, twice Nobel Prize winner who maintained that a mineral was the lowest common denominator to all illness or disease processes. This knowledge has been written about since the 1930s. It's very hard to understand how such basic knowledge is rarely taken into account to benefit human health, excepting by the mineral therapist.

While attending Melbourne's naturopathic college, I worked part-time in various naturopathic clinics. Modalities of treatment included herbs, homeopathics, vitamins and minerals. People paid a small fortune but because their health improved they kept coming. But it was not until I worked for Les Fisher that I found he used celloids exclusively, exactly as Maurice Blackmore had recommended, as a sole modality. No other practitioner in Melbourne used minerals alone, minerals with the pharmaceutical dose.

"But how can you expect results from so few remedies", I asked?

"How can I find out if someone returns without the expected results, where to look if I have prescribed a whole variety of medications. That's unscientific."

I asked Les one day if he thought there was a mineral compound particular to Australia. I expected him to say "magnesium phosphate." He said "calcium fluoride." I pondered on this and have come to see that quite apart from our tooth enamel there are connective tissue disorders like aneurisms, joint problems etc., but also when calcium fluoride becomes lacking in the arachnoid tissue round the brain, enough shrinkage occurs (not just pregnant women either) that we become more inflexible in our thinking. Mentally, calcium fluoride deficient people can also become somewhat parsimonious.

Les had gone from electrical engineering straight into studying naturopathy. He'd worked full time and attended the RMIT Melbourne 5 nights a week studying electrical engineering and was introduced to Blackmores minerals by a fellow worker. Les had carried extremely bad eczema and asthma from childhood and it was his experience with the celloids on himself that had led him to naturopathy. As a practitioner, he was always cautious and the second visit was made for two weeks later, when symptoms were already usually showing promise. He also advised patients to not alter other medications : to keep the status quo. It was unheard of in other naturopathic clinics in Melbourne at that time, where patients were told to wait at least three months for signs of improvement.

At this stage I did not think of becoming a naturopath myself, although I studied for my diploma but could not tear myself away from these positive experiences and it became more and more important to me to find out how real all of this was. Besides the college, I found it surprising that such a health industry was blooming in Melbourne, when it seemed stagnant in London, in Europe and in the two big U.S. cities I'd explored. When I left Brisbane in 1960 there was only the Sanitarium Health Shop.

In 1970, Maurice Blackmore's Food Remedy book was available to health shops all over Australia, the first of its kind to offer health education free of charge to the general public, particularly about minerals and foods richest in them. Maurice Blackmore was a man of many parts who devoted his life to the benefit of other Australians. My memoir will be my evidence of the profound truth Maurice Blackmore bequeathed to us and great thinkers before him like Dr William Schussler, reputedly the father of biochemistry and Noble prize winning scientist, Linus Pauling.

Maurice Blackmore maintained that practitioners should always think of the gut, where most chronic health problems started. If the ph balance is out, either due to poor diet and/or extreme stresses, often sodium phosphate is required to restore the ph balance. It is interesting today that modern medicine is exploring the value of good gut bacteria, when this has been known and observed by naturopaths for decades, yet without addressing the ph balance, the good gut bacteria may not survive. Modern medicine is very worried about the areas of medicine where Australian health is worsening. Today we have been told we have the worst allergy problems in the world.

Allergy problems can be tricky, even with the correct use of the minerals, but those who persist can gain health they may never have experienced, like a lady who has just collected her two mineral combinations, one that cleanses the allergens from the body and the other that addresses the ph balance and nervous system. Even on all the medicines she had been taking, her life had been a misery. Now she says she no longer needs the antihistimines and is thinking of giving up the Losac she said she was taking for excessive stomach acidity. Her diet had been extremely limited, but last Christmas she ate all the Christmas food with little reaction. She says she will be happy to take the minerals forever, as she never thought she would enjoy life as much as she does now.

My memoir will also tell the story of how essential minerals lacking in soils and processed foods reveal particular lacks in populations where I have lived and worked. More alarmingly, science is raising the question of increasing levels of CO2 interfering with the uptake of minerals by our plants, when over 80% of our foods come from plants which convert the minerals from the soil into what's best absorbed by us. One researcher finds that plants are filling up with sugar as percentages of minerals are left in the soil. I first read of this CO_2 phenomenon in the New Scientist in November 2002, in an article called Plague of Plenty.

If we do not understand how the mineral elements activate the very processes of life, we cannot see that quite apart from climate change, we should severely reduce atmospheric CO_2 to keep the balance in our atmosphere. Atmospheric scientist James Lovelock has written (Gaia, Allen & Unwin, 1991) that over a period of 3.6 billion years, Earth's homeostatic systems have kept steady Earth's temperatures by managing to keep down carbon dioxide levels. It's not just about climate change. Increasing levels of CO_2 may be progressively deleterious to the health of all species as we increasingly starve for essential elements of life, CO_2 inhibits the uptake of.

~ Three ~

LES FISHER'S PRACTICE AT
BEAUMARIS AND MENTONE.

What we learned from the 1970s, we owe to the courageous people with stubborn problems, often unresponsive to more conventional treatment who stuck with the minerals while progress was occurring, even when that progress seemed uneven at first. It dawned on us as time went by that when specific symptoms were provided for, the healing capacity seemed to increase more and more, but in the order of healing dictated by Nature.

It is Les Fisher's practice in Beaumaris first, then Mentone that I shall write about as he was the only practitioner who prescribed the minerals as a sole modality. His patients were a mixture of people and often professional, university and business people. In other practices were I worked, the patients were usually working class people and they were prescribed many different preparations, including herbs, homeopathic remedies etc. The cost to the patient with Les was therefore considerably lower and already within the first two weeks, improvements were observed by the patient and practitioner.

It was fascinating and also a little frightening that patients arrived with such an array of chronic and seemingly intractable problems.

It was in 1972 that I remember perhaps the first monumental case, which was of a middle-aged woman with pustular psoriasis all over her body. She said the skin specialist told her that hers was the worst case he had ever seen. She was put in an oxygen tent naked for months. Later, if she went into a restaurant, people walked out. I remember the psoriasis was particularly dense in her hair and on her hands. She developed the psoriasis following medical treatment with streptomyacin which had saved her life. Fortunately on the minerals, the psoriasis seemed to clear up completely, but sometime later I ran into her and her husband in a coffee shop and she said she was disappointed that she still needed to take some minerals because little patches of psoriasis sometimes reappeared. The lady's skin specialist rang Les Fisher about his treatment, but thought it was probably a fluke.

Years later in Tasmania, I treated a man whose psoriasis seemed to develop in a similar way to the lady in Melbourne. He was a big raw-boned Queenslander who had nearly killed himself on an icy Tasmanian winter road skidding to avoid a kangaroo in the early morning on his way to work. He crashed into a big tree on Sandfly Road and was so severely injured that when he recovered in hospital, he was told that had it been possible to locate his family, the life support systems would probably have been turned off. They did not expect him to live. Obviously the careful medical treatment saved his life, but as with the previous case, bad psoriasis developed. I saw him two years later when other treatment had not resolved the problem. Fortunately the skin healed completely on the minerals and I did not hear of any recurrence. As with the previous case, potassium sulphate was one mineral compound crucial to healing the skin.

Also around the same time in Melbourne, a woman came to see Les as she was supposed to have her gall bladder out. She was pregnant and she had three other children. She was terrified at the thought of surgery and took her minerals assiduously throughout the pregnancy, managing to avoid surgery. She gave birth at the local hospital. At lunch-time the midwife decided the birth was not imminent and went to lunch, though the mother thought the baby was about to be born. The baby was born almost immediately with the umbilical cord tight round its neck and stayed like that until the midwife returned. The baby was blue in the face and the mother was told the child was probably brain damaged. We saw the baby some months later. He looked like a skinny little rat with green mucous oozing from eyes, nose, mouth, every orifice. Les prescribed one mineral compound and suggested Roberts (a gritty unrefined) soy compound instead of a milk product. A few years later we were visited by the family. Looking at the children we saw immediately a child from whose face shone a quiet and very definite intelligence. This was the child whose mother had taken minerals throughout her pregnancy and despite the difficult start to life he had grown into a bright healthy looking little boy.

Another memorable child from the early seventies I'll call Phoebe. Phoebe's elder sister had asthma and her brother was swollen with fluid due to poor kidney function. Phoebe was worst off. She had stopped growing and digesting food. Medically nothing could be done and the child seemed to be dying.

For the first two months on the minerals her digestion and energy improved. Then the improvement suddenly stopped. Les then added Siberian ginseng for the next few months and the child again improved in growth and skills and became a happy, bubbly little person. Not having access to this record, I am writing from memory. I think Phoebe was 10 years old when Les saw her, but had not grown or developed beyond age 5 or 6. Her mother took her for her yearly appointment with the specialist. The specialist was delighted at the improvement, until the mother told him about the minerals. Then he got up, took the mother by her arm and ushered them out and closed the door after them. Phoebe stayed on the minerals, perhaps for a year while catching up on growth and development. We heard later that she got a job in a factory where she was very popular due to her happy nature. The last we heard, she had got married : all due to a courageous, determined mother and the elements of life.

Another memorable and quite humbling experience from the early 70s was a vivacious young Catholic girl whose ovulation had stopped when she was put on the pill in her early teens. Now she was a young woman in her twenties. She and her husband were wanting to have a baby. After months on the minerals, the symptoms that occurred instead of a period, i.e. migraine headaches, fluid retention and loss of hair no longer happened, but still her period did not come. Les Fisher told her he was taking her money under false pretences, as she was still not ovulating. She was laughing as she came out of the consulting room and said to me "I told him I was a good Catholic and I believe that if I stick to what I am doing I will ovulate eventually." Once again and the only other time this happened, Les added Blackmore's Siberian Ginseng to the minerals and refused to take payment for them. Months went by, then one day she rang and said she had the worst migraine she ever had, worse than anything previously. Les told her to chew up one magnesium phosphate tablet (65 mgs) with hot water and take hourly. Next day the migraine had gone, but she had swelled up with fluid, again worse than before after no swelling at all for months and she took sodium sulphate (195 mgs) hourly. The next day she ovulated and a month later she conceived. She had a beautiful happy daughter who was champion runner in her school, became an engineer and today is married with a family of her own. The girl this story is about, together with her husband had been told by a top Melbourne gynaecologist to adopt, that they would never have a child naturally. (This was before IVF). In the end they had three children.

Les treated a German woman who could no longer snow ski due to severe rheumatoid arthritis. Once she was skiing again she got her husband to come who had digestive problems if I remember rightly. The husband did well and invited Les to talk at a meeting of CEDA (Committee for Economic Development of Australia). This man was managing director of a large German company. I think he was a bit disappointed at Les' talk and so was I. But those early years were overwhelming and Les was still unsure about results that were often astounding and so at variance to our understanding about how the body could heal with only a little regular significant help.

One day he overheard me tell someone that I thought he could successfully treat a particular problem. Later he said to me "You have put me under great pressure. I don't always get good results with that problem. You don't realise what an effort the accuracy required means." So I went and checked the patient record cards and was able to point out that the consistently good results came with those who religiously took the tablets as prescribed. The best patients in fact were often the ones who started with the worst problems.

Les treated another woman who had been quite debilitated with arthritis. After some months when she was a lot better she asked Les if he could help her husband. Her husband was not expected to survive the winter with severe emphysema and he was a heavy smoker. Les was always prepared to try, even if at first it seemed impossible. This frail, wizened little man somehow survived the winter. Then he gave up smoking and went back to repairing fine clocks and watches, which he had not done for 17 years. Christmas came. We were on holidays and so was this man's doctor. He got the flu. He was given a penicillin injection by the locum doctor and he was allergic to penicillin and died. His wife was heartbroken. She had expected him to die from the emphysema. Yet he was recovering and looking so much better. It was a bitter blow.

One morning a woman rang me in great distress. She said no one could help her and she had been sent home from hospital to die. She had a huge hiatus hernia which would rise up and choke her so could not sleep at night. She had recently been surgically opened up and told she was like perished India rubber inside, so stitches were out of the question. "Please don't tell me you can help me if you can't!" I told her one could not tell if her body tissues might heal, but she would find out within the first weeks if there was any improvement. I will never forget her. She looked like someone from a concentration camp, nothing but bone and sunken black eye sockets. She'd had 27 years of digestive disorders. At first she could only hold down a little yoghurt, Roberts soy compound and after a few weeks, a little mashed vegetable. To our amazement she slowly got better on her crushed minerals and warm water. In those days Blackmores were allowed to make a 2 mg calcium fluoride tablet and that compound was essential. (Later calcium fluoride could only be made in a homeopathic dose. Apparently the Health Department thought it might be too much with fluoride medicating us all in our water supply, even though the fluoride in our water was not calcium fluoride which is required by all the connective tissue in our bodies). She developed small firm breasts, miraculous from her previous flat figure and became very interested in recipe books. She was 45 years old when she started the minerals which she took for many months and returned to the minerals later, when problems appeared, such as recurring staph ear infections. Years later she got in touch following house renovation and heavy lifting and painting the ceiling. She now lived in country Victoria and sent for the minerals as needed which fortunately she responded to despite occasional bouts of digestive problems. It was good to know that she enjoyed at least two more decades of happy, relatively healthy living. We've only lost touch in the last few years.

A former bank manager who had twice experienced a bank hold-up became a patient, because he had lost his nerve and suffered great debility after being held twice at gun-point and could not work. Within some months his nervous system had improved greatly and he was able to return to work. Since studying Psychology at university I've learned the value of cognitive behavioural therapy, but if a person becomes extremely debilitated, such exercises can cause more distress, if the person feels worse after doing them. However once they build up on the minerals if their metabolisms show the need, they can at last benefit from CBT, if still required.

A woman came to see us whom we had seen some years previously when Les practised in Mentone. He had moved his clinic to Frankston. She and other family members had been treated successfully with the only minerals Les would use with the balance of the cation/anion relationship (the positive and negative charge, as originally understood by doctors of biochemistry. - more later). This woman was exhausted and her husband had to drive her to the appointment. "I want to go on a cruise in two months and I can't go as I am now" she said. A month later she drove herself for the next appointment. She responded quickly and was able to enjoy her cruise. She had been prescribed mineral orotates by a local doctor. These minerals are usually much stronger in dose than Les used and did not observe the cation/anion relationship, which respects the action of the anion, the negative charge to determine the action of the cation, or positive charge. Larger doses of minerals can further exhaust a person. We don't have to slug our biochemistry to encourage it to function better.

I hesitated to put in this story in case someone thought I was claiming a cancer cure, but it deserves to be written about due to the great courage of this man and his family. Not everyone who has the bone pointed at them will die (the Aborigine tradition of pointing the bone which seemed to lead to the death of the person the bone was pointed at). One day a man and his wife arrived, recommended from a fellow student from the naturopathic college. He was medically diagnosed with terminal cancer. He had been opened up and the cancer was also in the spleen, so they were advised to have a last good holiday. Les said to me after seeing him "That man should not have got cancer." "Where was the weakness?" I asked. Les said that his diet was quite good and he swam before work each morning but he thought the weakness was in his nervous system. He was managing/director of a big insurance company. Months went by and after many months, the cancer could not be found. Then his wife had a nervous breakdown. She had expected her husband to die. So she was also treated on the minerals. Then it came his daughter's wedding and her father was able to give her away and he also went back to work in the same job he had had to leave. Just before we left to go to Hobart to live, the man arrived with a sinus problem. He had now retired from work and was in tears when he learned that Les was moving. Over those years there had been no recurrence of cancer. This man was a gentleman in every sense of the word and I feel privileged to have this story to write.

I should add that people do not come to me to treat their cancer, but will come if they are having a lot of pain and depression with the medical treatment and they will come when treatment is finished to rebuild their health, to try to lessen the weakness that lead to the cancer in the first place.

There are so many experiences from these years that I'm trying to keep to the most memorable and also am trying to write about a great range of conditions Les treated : and we learned that almost irrespective of the condition, when symptoms for minerals were there, the person would benefit and health would improve.

One day a man came for an appointment who I remembered from when I had first become receptionist/secretary. "Have you had a recurrence of your previous symptoms?" I asked. He stared at me and said shortly, "No. This is entirely different". He was right and did not require the original many months of treatment. This experience made me realise, that despite some years of observing such unexpected healing, I had not really believed what I saw. Then I remembered my work friends at Pan Am who could not believe that a big city like London was not dangerous at night. It can take time for change in perceptions to occur and I am so worried about how increasing CO_2 may be robbing us of the elements of life, that I only hope there is time for investigation and change for us to help the continuance of life. I've realised that without necessary levels of minerals in plants and all creatures we can eventually expect life to cease.

Another great learning experience was from a suffering child and her courageous mother. This skinny little girl had been sent by a doctor to Les, as he decided he was not helping her. This was in 1982. I was pregnant and some months later left the practice. The child was covered in eczema so badly that her arms were always covered in long sleeves. Skin conditions make me nervous. It seems that the skin, being the outer organ gets only what's left of the minerals and apart from daily requirements, there's also growth spurts for children. That's another way of saying that progress did not occur as we were used to seeing. In fact, when I left work I used to pray for help for this dear little girl. We meanwhile had moved to Tasmania and it was some years later that I visited Les' clinic in Frankston that he had retained. I was standing in the waiting room and a woman with a beautiful teenage girl came in. The girl had eyes sparkling with health. The mother said to me "You do not recognise my daughter do you?" and she said her name. I could not believe it!! Surely this beautiful girl could not be the wretched, skinny child I remembered. "But she did not get better on the minerals. Why did you stick to them?" "Because we found she was better on them than off them. Then one day I said to her, Simone, let's stop the cortisone cream. We had tried unsuccessfully once early on when she started the minerals. I don't think it's really helping you any more. So we stopped it. Then some time later she was about to start high school and the uniform had short sleeves. We wondered what we'd do. Suddenly, the week-end before she was due to start high school, the eczema vanished completely and she has never got it back." I am still in tears as I write this true story. I see that little girl and the radiant beauty she became. The question is, if one is topping up growing children trying to overcome deficits, can one expect these years of added minerals to help provide a firmer foundation for life as a healthy, untroubled teenager and adult?

One day my cousin rang up from Sydney. His son was in the Junior New South Wales Volleyball team. He was in great pain with his back. He was diagnosed with severe Scheuermann"s Syndrome and was told he would never play volleyball again and he was devastated. "Can your minerals help him", my cousin asked? Les prescribed three different celloid combinations. We were unsure as to the degree they"d help him. I think he took them for about six months. Some months later we learned that he'd won a sports scholarship to a U.S. university, where he played volleyball in the university team. He studied sports medicine and returned to Australia to become captain of the Australian Volleyball Team. Today he's a very successful business man. I checked with his family before including this story and they were very favourable. This retired champion still cares about his health. It's a shame that in an age of sports medicine, the elements of life our bodies require for all activities is largely ignored. We need the minerals in Nature's cation/anion relationship, which cannot be patented, but combinations that can be patented, cannot be expected to rebuild the body as occurs naturally when the minerals are optimal and in doses and formats as close as possible to how Nature requires them.

One interesting thing we observed during those years in Melbourne in the 1970s was that young children who came to the clinic and who had been treated with ongoing courses of antibiotics, seemed to benefit from the minerals instead of antibiotics, with their new adult teeth that came through. Whereas the baby teeth may have been mottled and discoloured, the new teeth that came through while they took minerals for their health problems were strong and white and I heard that these children often avoided the need for orthodontic treatment later as the jaw bones grew to support the teeth without overcrowding.

Les loved animals and treated dogs and cats, so I'll finish this chapter with the story of Rory and a stray cat before writing about the politics of the 70s and the double-blind trial at the Austin Hospital in 1977.

Rory was Australia's champion Irish setter for 7 years in a row. His owners had got very run-down with all the dog shows and I think there were a few health problems too. As they got better, they wondered if anything could be done for Rory. He had become listless and lost weight. He was getting progressively weaker and the vet had not succeeded in helping him. Les told the woman that her mineral tablets might also help Rory. So that night she gave Rory one each of her tablets at bedtime. At 4.00 a.m. Rory bounded onto their bed, which was the first time in many months. It had been his habit to make an early morning leap on to their bed. Some weeks later they brought this magnificent animal to see us. He really was quite unforgettable.

Dogs with arthritis often respond quickly too. I remember one who went on the minerals, got better, then gradually deteriorated again. One dose of his previous minerals and he was off rabbiting again, after the first dose. I'm glad to say later in Tasmania, a dog referred to me got run over and was going to lose his back leg. On the minerals he made quite a quick recovery and the damaged leg seemed as good as new.

We were living at Dromana when a stray white cat with sun damaged ears and nose appeared. The cat was irritable. Les fed it. We were surprised when it was there in the morning. Les picked it up and it tried to scratch him. It was burning hot. He put it in a box with a blanket and got some minerals down its throat. Then it broke out in lice all over its body, so more minerals and Les carried it outside to do its business and it slept in its box by our bed. Its back leg swelled up and broke open on the outside and a huge amount of pus came out. Then the same leg, still swollen opened on the inside and more pus came out. It had lots of doses of minerals like potassium sulphate. Once the two openings were no longer excreting pus, they healed up quickly. It amazed us that the perforations disappeared completely - no scarring. You could see no sign of where the skin had opened. The cat got better - no lice, no fever and it seemed well. Then it went bush and we never saw it again. To us it was an unforgettable lesson in how nature can heal with only the help of the elements of life.

~ Four ~

POLITICS, EDUCATION AND DOUBLE BLIND TRIAL AT AUSTIN HOSPITAL.

In the mid 1970s a board of 5 professors was set up by Gough Whitlam's government to investigate the practices of Chiropractic, Osteopathy and Naturopathy. These professors were allocated a year for their investigation and during this year, Les Fisher appeared before them twice and was then invited to a luncheon in Sydney, together with executives of Blackmores Laboratories. At this lunch, Professor Rand of Melbourne challenged Les over lack of scientific evidence regarding the mineral modality Les used in practice. Les argued back about the impossibility of his situation to organise such a trial within medicine. In fact, the regulations within the National Health Act had to be changed at a federal and state level to allow Les, a non-medical person, to conduct research in a teaching hospital setting. Professor Webb, who had heard the exchange between Professor Rand and Les Fisher agreed that Les could not do the research without their help.

Professor Rand had a student who needed a research project towards her Ph.D. There was only six months left for the professors to complete their investigation, so they hurriedly chose Behavioural Problems with Children and some children, whom the Austin Hospital found unresponsive were put into a crossover double-blind trial, set up with active mineral and/ or placebo tablets. Both were coloured white and supplied by Blackmores Laboratories. At the end of the 6 month trial, the children were assessed by doctors, parents, teachers and Les Fisher, the prescribing practitioner. There were EEG results before and after, which were not published, as this was the last study of the investigation and had to be rushed to meet the year deadline, but the electroencephalogram results, like the trial results were significantly different and it was suggested that further trials should be conducted (Webb Report, Government Archives, Swanston Street, Melbourne, 1977).

After the trial, some of the parents brought their children across the city to continue treatment on the minerals until a level of behavioural stability was attained.

During the early 1970s behavioural problems in children became a gradually accepted term to describe children who had become uncontrollable in schools. During my own childhood, problems teachers were now being faced with, with occasional uncontrollable children were almost non-existent. If you were naughty and talked too much, you went and stood outside the door. Of course during the 1950s our food had been grown without chemical soil stimulants and foods were not preserved. By Monday at school, the bread our sandwiches were made of had become stale. We were so glad when the week's fresh bread arrived.

In America in the 1960s I was horrified that sugar was put in bread and was tasteless, despite the sugar and bread and milk never seemed to go off, unlike the fresh foods I was used to in England and Australia at that time. Is it a coincidence that as foods became preserved for market economy, behavioural problems also were developing in children? We do know that food processing reduces mineral and vitamin content in food.

At that time, in the 1970s, some schools like private schools would not tolerate disruptive children. One boy we treated was an only child who had lost his father in a car accident and his mother too had been badly injured. He attended an expensive prestigious school from which he was expelled. His mother was determined to help him become more stable. So he was put on the minerals. After many months, he had settled down well and won a scholarship to a Melbourne University, though he was well under age and later won a scholarship to an American university, again under age. These children often seemed to me to be highly intelligent. Les agreed and quoted Maurice Blackmore and his idea about "the missing links."

Years later, when I was in Tasmania, I believe it was Time magazine that had a short article "Is it Nature or Nurture" about people who had grown into monsters. I decided it was both nature AND nurture. Children who were destructive and might grow into destructive adults were lucky if, like those I had known, they had mothers who would support them through outgrowing behavioural problems with the essential nutrients the body requires from the minerals. One beautiful little girl I remember was so violent she would smash windows, mirrors or anything nearby and attack her parents with knives and did not sleep at night. Life was hell for the family. particularly the mother who the doctor was inclined to blame. I found the original patient record card and rang and fortunately the mother answered the phone. She said her daughter, now in her late twenties was fine as long as she got enough sleep. She asked me for Les Fisher's phone number. The terrible problems were a thing of the past. So I wrote back to the magazine and said it is Nature, when one addresses the basic biochemistry and it is Nurture when a wonderful parent, often the mother saw to the developing child's needs. Of course my letter was not published.

The children themselves learned to avoid foods that triggered bad behaviour for days afterwards. So at parties, they often avoided soft drinks and highly coloured cordials and cakes full of sugar. Often the children stayed on the minerals for months. They were stopped when the children seemed normal. Then behaviour might become erratic again following a growth spurt and they would need topping up with the minerals for a few months and this might go on until puberty when things seemed finally to consolidate.

One three-year old I have remembered was a miserable little monster who would come in and wipe his snot on the curtains and often get bored while waiting, so scream the place down. He did not respond quickly. With other children, we were used to the behaviour of the child responding first, even before the asthma, eczema etc. the child was receiving treatment for and with older children, the teacher commenting on the child's co-operation and good behaviour in class, all within the first weeks of being on the minerals. A neighbour told me that this particular child lived on ice cream and coca cola and refused everything else, so she didn't see how he would get over his bronchial problems. His mother gave into him. So I asked the mother what he would eat and drink that would do him any good. She was very worried because he had put on no weight for a year. In the end she thought he might like pineapple juice (refused all vegetables and fruit), so I got her to agree to give him nothing but unsweetened pineapple juice with a little brewers yeast with its protein, minerals and vitamins for a week and his minerals. He put on over a kilo of weight in that week. After that the mother had the confidence to try him on other foods which he then became more cooperative with and he soon got better.

It was because of children responding in behaviour and wellbeing first, that Les had the confidence to do the double-blind trial at the Austin Hospital. Of course we encouraged better diet in the clinic and I was concerned about results from the trial with only the minerals. Les said to me "Do you think the often exhausted mothers worry about the diet before their child gets results from the minerals?"

One boy who came to the clinic from the double-blind trial was a young teenager. He resented being dragged along, but because he was better on the minerals, his mother insisted. Then months later they arrived and he had a big smile on his face. He had just been offered an apprenticeship he was very pleased about. It was good to see the resentment had vanished at last.

Also during the 1970s, educational standards were improving at both the naturopathic and chiropractic colleges in Melbourne. Les was a lecturer at the naturopathic college and when Janus Fawke from the Chiropractic College began seeking a standard of regulation for government registration, Les joined him for meetings with Mr Rossiter, Victoria's Health Minister, Mr Roper ALP and Mr Ross-Edwards, Country Party at meetings at the

Windsor Hotel in Melbourne. Jan Fawke thought that naturopaths could also gain registration along with chiropractors. But time was now short and the chiropractors had acquired excellent college premises and established a solid science teaching basis. Jan Fawke suggested that in the interim, naturopaths might gain registration by sharing the college premises and basic science teachers, allowing students to continue after basic science subjects in either stream of chiropractic or naturopathy.

Les was delighted with this offer to take back to the naturopathic college where Alfred Jacka was college dean. But Alf Jacka thought naturopathy would be taken over by chiropractic and encouraged the students and the few naturopaths who attended the meeting to discuss the proposal, that it should be vetoed. Les Fisher and Peter Van Wunnik who practised in Coburg, thought that such an opportunity for registration of naturopaths might not come again "A once in a lifetime opportunity" said Les.

In 1978 chiropractors became registered as Doctors of Chiropractic. Les, Peter Van Wunnik and one naturopathic student, John Froelich chose to study for chiropractic registration and became Doctors of Chiropractic. Academic courses were conducted at the Preston Institute of Technology, where Les Fisher later taught.

Meanwhile in 1975, Les and I took a holiday to Denmark, where we have wonderful friendships among the happiest natured, most generous unforgettable people and to England. I remembered from living in London, that there were still threads of natural medicine to be found, (not like we had in Melbourne) and there was an Osteopathic college off Baker Street. I said to Les "They need the celloids here. Do you think it would be possible to set up a seminar?" We were a week in London and Les introduced himself at the osteopathic centre and was able to interest them in an introductory celloid seminar.

On our return to Australia, Les told Marcus Blackmore (Maurice Blackmore's son, who was now managing/director of Blackmores Laboratories), what he had organised in London and Blackmores agreed to pay for the seminar. From that first seminar, Les organised the importing and distribution to be run by Kenneth Roberts, an osteopath from Eastbourne, who became a very good friend over the coming years. Every year Les went to London to conduct a week-end seminar. I went with him and we also went to Denmark. Practitioners traveled from all over the British Isles, including the Queen's physician, a homeopathic physician (Queen Elizabeth is known to have taken homeopathic remedies for decades and look at her astounding good health and work output). They had a week-end seminar presented by Les and the third day was for discussion of practitioner problems and successes. In 1991 there were several hundred new and returning practitioners at Les' final mineral seminar in London at one of the Hilton Hotels.

Les lectured for Blackmores from 1976 to 1993. He also took his celloid educational programme to South Africa, Hong Kong, Ghana and New Zealand. Mineral therapy is still thriving in New Zealand as well as Australia. While he was away, I looked after the practice. I had my diploma, but Les worked as a sole practitioner and I worked supportively and learned. Les was a thorough, inspirational teacher.

Meanwhile in Melbourne, Les treated his patients with celloids and when their problems were resolved, they were recom-

mended to their local health shop where they could buy Blackmores mineral compounds, vitamins etc. to maintain their
health. Blackmores business in health shops increased to the
point where Rodney and Lowella Brennan were appointed as
Blackmores Victorian distributors. Blackmores business grew
fast in Victoria during the years Les practised there. Years later
in Tasmania, Blackmores had a wonderful representative called
Wendy Purtell. She broadcast my successes all over the state. I
spoke to practitioners she put me onto and again Blackmores
mineral business grew fast. The same thing happened with Les
Fisher's Active Elements in Tasmania. I used them. Others heard
and began using them too.

Meanwhile Les and I had married and our daughter was born in
1983. I stayed home with her and I did the banking from home.
One evening, I attended a meeting at the Mechanics Institute in
Frankston where CSIRO scientist, Barry Pittock introduced his
book The Nuclear Winter. My baby was home with her father
and I was horrified to learn that within a week, nuclear war
in the northern hemisphere would spill its nuclear waste over
to the southern hemisphere. I was and still am against producing technology we cannot neutralise the waste from. From this
meeting, where for the first time I publicly spoke, I was asked
to be press officer for the Dunkley branch of the Australian Democrats and for a few years wrote regularly in the Mornington
Peninsula newspapers and what I learned went into my letters
to the press.

Then bank interest rates went up rather suddenly. Les believed
we had fixed interest on our mortgage. Our interest had not altered, then suddenly went up to nearly 18 per cent. Les went

immediately to the bank manager who pointed out a few words finely printed on the bottom line of the agreement. We had friends in Tasmania who were trying to sell a 50 acre block of land, only 13 km from Hobart, so suddenly we were interested. I took our little toddler Juliet with me and I was thrilled at this land surrounded by hills, that reminded me of where I had grown up on the edge of Brisbane. Here our little girl could have the natural life I had enjoyed as a child. So we moved to Tasmania.

~ Five ~

HOBART AND A NEW
PRACTICE.

Hobart was so different. First of all, we were Mainlanders which seemed to me worse than foreigners. We loved our land and our beautiful house, built with sandstone/concrete blocks and an Italian terracotta roof. The builder had to get an Italian roof tiler and his son over from Melbourne to do the roof. We had blackwood benches, and a wonderful sassafras staircase, tanks in ground and an access road nearly 1 km long, including a bridge over a gully all of which needed maintaining, particularly after rain. Les kept his clinic, in the State Bank building in Frankston, travelling to and from Melbourne. He bought a little flat in Frankston. We had lived in Mt Eliza and Saturday morning meant a visit to a coffee shop. But there were none in Hobart, not until the Retro at Salamanca Place opened in 1992.

Very soon Les decided that Hobart was a good place to retire to ; not to set up a practice like his. He wrote another textbook for Blackmores, then took the opportunity to become Company secretary for Blackmores U.K. Meanwhile Juliet our daughter was school age and I found the only job I could get with World Book, travelling round country roads. Les already had a few patients and he said that with my naturopathic diploma, I could take over his practice while he went to England. I wanted to go too and what about Juliet!! In the end I managed with help on the land from a good man called Lin Jacobson who worked for the Hydro. He cut wood for us and himself, made paddocks for his horses and Juliet's pony and maintained the access road when needed.

We sent Juliet to Friends School which I could not maintain when Les left. I was very nervous practising with no one to refer to. It amazed me how people found out where I was and would visit me arriving off the primitive access road at the other end of which our neighbour bred racehorses.

The first patient had been referred to Les by a local doctor but Les had gone. He was a builder who had been in hospital for 6 weeks with diarrhoea which had still not stopped. That first consultation had taken an hour. I sent him home with a few minerals and he was to take them that night and four times next day and to ring me the following morning. When he rang, he said "I suppose you know what I am going to say". I did not and was worried sick. He said he had his first partial bowel motion next morning and this morning, a complete bowel motion. He was very pleased and I felt lucky. Diarrhoea can be caused by so many things, but his diet had remained fairly bland. He was not contributing to it, so the minerals helped quite quickly.

We had only been on the land a couple of weeks and a neighbour was gathering wood into a trailer with a friend of his. I went up to say hello. Our neighbour said his friend was very sad as his wife was pregnant and had been told she would lose her baby because of placental insufficiency and she was more than halfway through her pregnancy. I told them about the minerals and that the macro mineral tablets such as potassium, magnesium, calcium phosphates with sodium phosphate for the pH balance (promoting the healthy gut bacteria) may help the natural development of the growing baby. The prospective father said he would get his wife to try the minerals which I collected from the house. Many years later I was getting petrol when a motor mechanic from the garage came up to me. He was the prospective father from nearly 20 years ago. He said "Thank you for my beautiful, healthy daughter. My wife's pregnancy immediately improved when she took the minerals and she had a lovely baby girl." I said to myself a little prayer of thanks.

I was very lucky because word got around quickly and a steady trickle of people arrived up the access road. They were often people with stubborn problems that were not improving. One man had emphysema. He was one of many from the Huon and he took the minerals through a long, difficult winter and fortunately got better. Since then I have treated many members of his family and extended family. To my knowledge he has had no more minerals. I have heard he gets bronchial troubles often in the winter but so far is still here.

It was so different from Melbourne. After some months I noticed that often people came for a few months and then not a word. So after a few months later I started ringing people to find out how they were getting on. All of them said they had done well, though one said at first nothing had changed then suddenly her health problems went all at once. One lady had a history of sarcoidosis for which she had been treated with corticosteroids for many months. That was 10 years earlier, but she still had distressing symptoms. I asked if she had continued with the minerals and she said she had. "But you never really got better on them" I said. "Yes, but I am better on them than off them". I should have asked her where she got them as she was not seeing me. Years later I found that both the local pharmacy and health shop got them in. I have to say for the Tasmanians. They are an enterprising lot. Minerals were unheard of in Hobart when we arrived, but once people got benefit, interest grew quietly and fast.

There were so many different people and fascinating. One very elegant woman I shall never forget arrived in her expensive car, came in and said "I have high blood pressure. I have just tipped all my medication down the sink and I expect you to help". I had an immediate vision of the front page of the Mercury (Hobart's newspaper) "Naturopath responsible for Stroke". This woman was elegantly and expensively dressed and travelled interstate, sometimes more than once a week. She had a very high powered job which she loved. Her iris showed the open, holey texture of a poor constitution, but she had the initiative of a highly intelligent racehorse type. I prescribed the minerals according to her specific symptoms and to be taken 6 times daily until the blood pressure stabilised, then worried myself sick for a week, but fortunately she responded. The pressures of her job meant she had to take very regular doses of minerals. Input needs to balance output. Eventually she married and decided to retire from work and play golf. The last time I saw her she was as elegant as ever and so much more relaxed than originally.

I treated people from the Dutch Reform Church in Kingston. A woman came to see with a stubborn infectious problem. She was greatly debilitated. She named her condition which I can't remember, but then we naturopaths don't treat disease, we treat according to specific symptoms of the patient, then trust the body will heal itself. She got better and then recommended me to a very beautiful young Dutch Australian mother with pure golden hair, two beautiful blonde little girls and her baby boy was the patient. He was two months old and had a shunt put in his brain for hydrocephalus. His skin was grey alabaster. The mother said he was discharged from hospital and she had been given no advice at all. I wished Les was there, but it was down to me. Over months the dear little boy became healthy and sturdy and I can still see him climbing the sassafras staircase. I still hear from this lady who has herself become a professional person and I am grateful that I have been trusted with her children's health over the years.

One day a mother rang me from the Royal Hobart Hospital . She said she was taking her little girl out because they were going to give her blood bodies. Her white blood cell count was extremely low. They had kept her there hoping her white blood count would build over the next few days. This did not happen. The hospital would not let the child leave without a crash helmet on her head. She could not afford to hit her head. I was very nervous about treating this child, but the mother was adamant. I gave her the particular mineral combinations I thought the child needed for her blood and lymphatic system and taking no chances, also gave her vitamin C with the bioflavinoids. It was the end of the week and on the Monday, the child was to return to the hospital for more tests. On the Sunday afternoon, the child had taken off the helmet and banged her head on a bed post. She came up in a big lump. but amazingly no bruising. The Royal Hobart Hospital monitored the child over the next week, while the white cell level normalised. I was reminded of this story by the child's father. He came to see me recently with a stubborn skin condition, and said he came because of how his youngest daughter was helped all those years ago. He said she was now studying at a university on the Mainland.

One girl who came to see me worked as a professional cleaner. She said she was allergic to everything and if she went to lunch with her friends, there was nothing she could eat without a bad reaction. After a few months she could go to lunch and no longer react to everything, so life had improved. Then she broke out in a boil below her breast. It was a recurring boil that had been treated with antibiotics and she was always left with a hard band where the boil had been. I told her that if she went with the minerals, it would go much slower, but she chose to do this rather than more antibiotics. After many weeks, the boil had gone and this time there was no more hard band where previous boils had been. Years later she went to Queensland and rang me one day about a friend's problem. "What about that boil you used to get" I asked her? "What boil" she said? She had forgotten all about it.

Another young woman was pregnant and sick all through the pregnancy even with the minerals. She had suffered ill health all her life yet at university she achieved highly when she did her degree, won a scholarship and this was despite her constant ill health. She was a very bright woman who was determined to gain good health. I think that during the pregnancy the baby got the benefit of the minerals and it wasn't until after the birth that her health started to build up. Despite increasing good health, she was still bedridden if she had a sliver of onion or garlic and could not take even a tiny amount of sodium sulphate (needed for the health of the liver and kidneys and which she showed symptoms for). Her mother and grandfather also could not eat garlic or onion. So we stayed with the sodium phosphate (looking after the pH balance). She was no longer showing any ill health at all, so after months she decided to try a tiny piece of sodium sulphate tablet and again reacted immediately, but perhaps not quite as severely as before. So a week or so later she tried another tiny piece of sodium sulphate with a little less reaction, staying on her other minerals she was not ready to give up. She continued in this way until she was no longer reacting and today can eat garlic and onion quite normally. She still finds the minerals maintain better health for her. It is through courage and determination like this that we have gained the knowledge I am hoping to pass on now.

One little girl I treated had Osgood Schlatter disease. She took the minerals for many months and even during that time was in a brace. The next year her father came to see me with recurring flu. He said this daughter, who had previously been the most unhealthy had become the healthiest person in the family so he now wanted help for himself.

What began to interest me was that I was prescribing potassium in one form or another, usually potassium phosphate for nearly everyone I saw, particularly from down the Huon. This was different from Melbourne. I remembered Hedley from the naturopathic college in Melbourne and what he said about the Irish soil. One day I had a dark-haired, dark blue eyed business man (the Irish look) from the Huon sitting opposite me and I asked him if there were a lot of Irish descendants from the Huon region. He smiled and said to me "Let me tell you an old Irish saying from the Huon:" *"the tiredness has come over me"*. That is a classical potassium phosphate symptom when often cannot drag oneself out of bed of a morning and potassium sulphate when one crashes after lunch.

I decided to buy 50 olive trees to plant on my land, not thinking about how barren the soil was. However I went up to the quarry for some bags of crusher dust and got a printout of the mineral content in the rock dust I was buying. I was quite shocked to learn that there was no iodine in the crusher dust. On Saturday I went to the Salamanca market to buy organically grown vegetables from a Dutch Australian farmer. This man was reputed to restore dead unproductive soil into very fertile soil. I told him about the crusher dust and the lack of iodine. "I know that but what about potassium?" I said that there was potassium but the content was very low. "I'm going to get some. No matter what I do I cannot keep potassium in the soil."

A family arrived one day in a big Mercedes Benz. The older children were at Bond University on the Gold Coast. None of them had bad problems and as we discussed the various members of the family and their concerns, it came out that their mother used to collect seaweed to eat from the Derwent River near where they lived. So I asked how their health was at this time. They looked at each other and then said it was good so I asked why she had stopped. Then I explained that research had found that sea vegetables are at least 20 times richer in minerals than anything grown on land. Well the minerals get washed down to sea, don't they! I was advising everyone who came to see me to gather the seaweed after a storm and spread it over their vegetable patches so the minerals could release into the soil, while protecting growing plants from the sun (very powerful UV here in Tasmania).

There was an exhibition not long after we arrived at the end of 1987, of early paintings of life in Tasmania that fascinated me when I saw so many of Tasmanian Aborigines. They looked so robust and healthy, not weedy and spindly like the Mainland Aborigines. Sometime later I learned that Tasmanian Aborigines ate seaweed, so full of minerals essential for human health. No wonder they were so well muscled and glowing with health. So what the ancient soil lacked they made up for out of the sea : the intelligence of so-called primitive people.

We had only been in Tasmania a few months when I received a phone call from an old friend in Victoria. She said she had just had a hysterectomy. "What for?" I asked. "Oh you know me. I was flooding with the menopause change and wanted it over, but I've rung to tell you something. You know I've had the same gynaecologist for all my women's things and he said he had never seen anything like it. When he opened me up he could find no adhesions. He said if had not done all the previous surgeries himself, he wouldn't have believed it. There was no trace of scar tissue. You will remember that before each surgery I took the minerals, one container of each until they were finished - a month's supply. I thought you'd be pleased." I remembered that her children had been delivered by caesarian section and she had had an ectopic pregnancy in between.

She also told me that she had taken her six month old son to see Les because he had bronchial asthma and she hoped to avoid drugs. I was pregnant with Juliet and not in touch with things in the clinic at the time. She said she ground the minerals between two spoons and gave them to her baby three times daily. He got over the bronchial troubles and they never returned. Years later she recommended the minerals her son took to a man who was laying vinyl in her house whose eight year old son had chronic asthma which ruled their lives. His wife worked in a chemist shop and found they dealt with the company which produced the tablets. The chemist said they would not hurt the child but probably not do any good either. About six months later the man knocked on her door and gave her a bouquet of flowers, a bottle of champagne and chocolates. He said "Thank you. The minerals have changed our lives and our son has not had an asthma attack since." My friend said that neither her doctor nor The Royal Children's Hospital, Melbourne were interested.

Just as well we live in Australia with an even more robust democracy than in Europe. In Europe the EU Codex law means that natural products are treated like prescription drugs. My understanding is that the law precludes the sale of vitamins etc., excepting in very low doses, without a prescription. As European doctors, like Australian doctors are taught relatively little natural medicine, it is no wonder that there is not the burgeoning health market in Europe that we still have access to in Australia. Our taxes pay an enormous medical bill for all Australians. Just imagine how much higher it might be if we could not help ourselves!

My friend's story reminded me of my first experience of treating a baby - my daughter. Juliet is very like her father and his family. Both his parents had histories of digestive problems and their son, her father had started life with bad colic. Juliet's grandfather was often rushed to hospital with bleeding stomach ulcers.

The minerals and a largely vegetarian diet meant that he lived into his nineties enjoying health he had not known as a younger man yet he smoked most of his life.

My baby screamed day and night with colic. At six weeks, the paediatrician said he'd be a rich man if he could find a cure for colic. He couldn't, so I must, at least that's what I thought in my exhausted state. So I powdered one potassium/magnesium phosphate tablet and one calcium/sodium phosphate tablet and gave them to my daughter in gripe water twice daily. Within two weeks the colic was gone and I decided to keep her on these two tablets two or three times daily through her childhood years. I took her off to Denmark to meet our wonderful friends. At five months she was a happy baby,

I was determined that she would not develop the eczema and asthma that marred the childhood of her father. When she was five she went through a growth spurt and for the first time eczema appeared on her arms, so I gave her three doses of minerals a day until the eczema cleared. About this time she went to the dentist who noted an occlusion on her front tooth but it had healed itself. It might be because of the molasses on a spoon I gave her, without cleaning her teeth. She never developed asthma or eczema and best of all is her still nearly perfect teeth, despite the weak tooth enamel she inherited. Her father's teeth had crumbled away by the time he was twelve. Juliet has had a baby herself (and took the minerals) and still has lovely teeth despite thin enamel. It's not only fluoride Australian soils lack, it's also calcium. We must have deteriorated as a people, because Australian soldiers who went to World War 1 had to have perfect teeth. Just as well that perfect teeth is not a pre requisite today or there would be hardly any soldiers.

My baby had not long recovered from colic and we were sleeping at last, when Les' secretary rang me one day. Les was lecturing in London and a patient had rang, a woman who was trying to get pregnant and had hoped to do so by taking the minerals for her symptoms to restore good health. "She is worried because her hormones are changing". So I asked for her telephone number and rang and asked the lady about her health. "There are no problems since I've been on the minerals, but my hormones are changing and I am 38. Perhaps I should go on IVF. " I told her that I had a new baby and was almost 42 and above all, with a new baby one needs one's health. I suggested she stay on the minerals for another 2 or 3 months, during which time, as her periods had changed, she may conceive naturally. She agreed to this plan. Later I heard that she conceived soon after our conversation and had a healthy baby boy. A few years later, the lady again got in touch with the clinic and said she now had had two healthy boys naturally and to please tell me.

I've treated women who had the symptoms of polycystic ovaries and other female problems. Once the terrible periods, often with huge clots no longer occur, a pregnancy may happen. It is as though nature does not want to overburden a person with an extra load. I often did not hear about the pregnancy, until a friend with similar problems was referred to me at the pharmacy where later I worked. It is amazing how basic biochemistry will restore health when all else has failed. Another almost epidemic concern today, following pregnancy is post natal depression. During the 1970s we rarely saw women with post natal depression, but again we found it responded well, when the woman's biochemistry was addressed.

One of my earlier patients at Kingston Downs, as we called our property was a woman who came to see me with severely depleted nerves. She had had 14 electric shock treatments and was rigid, almost catatonic and hissed through her teeth that she HATED her husband. Fortunately she responded better and better on the minerals and by the third visit told me about her wonderful husband and how much he did for her. Once she had become calmer and happier for some time, I did not see her again and I later heard that she had lived perhaps ten more years. I often wondered if she got minerals from the local chemist. I later found that she and the local chemist attended the same church. But she may have returned to conventional medicine. She was definitely another person who needed the potassium phosphate.

I saw people locally who had high blood pressure with other health problems. Some of them went to a doctor in Blackmans Bay who took them off their high blood pressure medication when their blood pressure had become normal over a period of time. Not every doctor will continue patients on medication when they no longer need it.

One family I shall never forget were a man and his children who had been subjected to heavy metal poisoning, the man saying he had "waded round in dieldrin and was exposed on the farm to aerial fallout from the nuclear explosions at Maralinga. Years later they moved to Tasmania where he became a craftsman, an artist in what he produced and now could no longer work and no one could help him. The family lived south of Huonville so it took over an hour to get to me in Kingston and the journey was so debilitating to him that he was bedridden for days after. Over months he became well enough to work again but one day he rang me distressed because a sudden weather change had brought a return of the terribly painful symptoms and he had to stop work. I explained that this would happen until a lot of toxins had cleared from his system.

Meanwhile, once her husband was responding, his very caring wife decided their 15 year old son should be treated. He had similar symptoms to his father. The son was at a school for children with severe learning difficulties. The son responded on the minerals quicker than his father. One day his mother said "He is now reading his letters together." I said, "What! Is he dyslexic?" "Severely dyslexic" said his mother. "He has been reading his numbers and letters upside down or back to front ". Then the 15 year old son said something I shall never forget. "What do you think it feels like to be told you will never be able to read or write?" His wonderful, persistent mother immediately had him doing remedial learning. He went from strength to strength, going to college then graduating in a field of fine craftsmanship which has provided an excellent career for him. I should not have been surprised that it was the learning abilities that responded first even though I had not prescribed with this in mind. We had seen so many children, where on the minerals they showed a need for, it was their behaviour, wellbeing and learning ability that improved first. The intelligence within our bodies prioritises. Meanwhile the family moved interstate but I saw the father again a couple of years ago with digestive problems he had been unable to resolve.

One day a patient told me that a naturopath who lived and practised a few miles from me, said to her that the celloids were
unnatural. I was surprised. Surely this naturopath had learned
about the beginnings of biochemistry with Dr William Schussler
and other European doctors? How could these minerals be unnatural when they are found in every cell of our bodies, other
animal bodies and plants we ingest them from? Perhaps he
thought the vegetables he recommended were replete in minerals ignoring increasing soil depletion, long storage and fruits
picked green etc. Because the celloids and other mineral combinations I recommend today are in the biochemical format,
where the positive charged mineral combines with a negative
charged mineral for specific purposes in the body, how can they
be considered unnatural and in this "natural" format, they cannot even be patented. In fact there is no medicine more natural
and they are very supportive to other kinds of medicine as medical doctors found when I later worked in pharmacies and local
doctors said they observed the benefits to their patients.

Meanwhile, while I saw people with a broad range of problems,
my daughter Juliet learned how to tame wild little Toby her
shetland pony. There was a Dutch Australian woman called Elizabeth who took children for a long week-end into her home and
taught them how to care for their horses. They took their sleeping bags and of course their horses. But we could not get Toby
onto the float, so Juliet went without her horse. On her return
she asked if she could have a riding lesson with Elizabeth. I rang
and Elizabeth said "Who?". I said "Juliet Fisher". "Well I am surprised. Juliet got into trouble a few times for being naughty, but
bring her by all means." Juliet rode Elizabeth's horse round a
corral heavily lined with sawdust while Elizabeth yelled instruc-

tions. Towards the end of the lesson, Elizabeth enthused as Juliet cantered round the oval, "She is brave. She will make a good rider". Juliet soon had naughty Toby in hand and rode him happily to pony club. On pony club Sunday, people rode their horses down from the hills, through our land, crossed the road and rode through the paddock opposite, on to pony club. Sometimes a little friend stayed overnight and the girls got up very early and polished their saddles and bridles and made everything perfect for next day when the horses and equipment would be carefully inspected. It was such wonderful training. We mothers brought the extras in our car boots and Juliet never forgot a thing. The children loved pony club.

In the late 1980s, minerals may not have been thought of in relation to human health, but there was a wonderful woman from Northern Ireland who made it her business to provide mineral rich nutrients in foods like molasses and kelp for the horses. She advocated advice from Pat Colby's horse book and everyone had a copy of this book including my daughter. We often saw her riding with others over the hills and sometimes through our land. It was so rural and now the hills are covered in housing estates as Kingborough is the fastest growing area in Tasmania.

In 1990 I enrolled at the University of Tasmania.

~ Six ~

UNIVERSITY AND A HORSE WITH COLIC AND A DOG WITH SNAKEBITE.

I was one of the mature aged students. Philosophy was one of the first year subjects I did and it taught me to think about my ideas more carefully. I was enthusiastic about philosophies that appealed to me and ignored what didn't. So I quickly learned about balance, to present arguments for and against. One subject was Free Will and Determinism. I believed in freewill much more then than now. Minerals and the years have taught me that Determinism prevails and that Free Will provides a flexibility, necessary for changing circumstances, but that it is actually an adjunct of Determinism. It never occurred to me then, that in learning how the mineral elements work and are essential to life's functions, I would develop a philosophy of my own, about the elements of life.

Psychology was another of my subjects which I followed through to a Master of Education degree in Counselling and Development. Another student who became a psychologist told me he did not understand why I was not intending to be a psychologist too. I told him that there were too few people practising as mineral therapists and why would I do this when I saw so many good results with the minerals. A few people who had been patients of mine, studied to become naturopaths but I still worried about the overall lack of knowledge and understanding. Some years later I sent a patient to this same psychologist as he also practised hypnotherapy. This is a later story with wonderful results.

I was also a member of the Hobart East Timor committee. Jennie Herrera kept us in touch with the dreadful political situation in East Timor and set up public speaking events. Michael Hodgman, father of Will Hodgman Tasmania's premier, often spoke at these meetings. This was before the East Timorese had voted to be independent from the invading Indonesians and the Australian media at last took an interest in the terrible brutality the East Timorese were subjected to following their election. I felt ashamed being Australian, because the East Timorese sometimes paid with their lives for protecting Australian soldiers from the Japanese during the second world war.

I wondered about Michael Hodgman, as he was in the Liberal Party and I said to him once "You wouldn't be too popular with the Liberal Party, speaking publicly for the East Timorese." He said he'd been told he wouldn't achieve much in his party because of this interest, but he had to live with his conscience. Many people have told me how he helped so many people when they needed legal advice. Each year when the A.L.P. had their annual conference at the Wrestpoint Casino, we made the delegates walk the gauntlet, past big coloured pictures of East Timorese atrocities they and the government were ignoring. We would not allow them to escape from the reality of what was happening in East Timor.

Towards the end of first year university, first year Arts students had some lectures in the Stanley Burbury Theatre. At the end of a lecture on South East Asia, the lecturer criticised Australian journalists for an unfair attitude to Indonesia which he said must change and then he asked for questions. I asked why he had not told the students about the murder of Australian journalists by Indonesian soldiers at Balibo, East Timor. Australian journalists were not just prejudiced, but were angered, because of an unjust, terrible fate to our journalists at the time of the Indonesian invasion, that was still ignored by our government all these years later in 1990.

Of course I talked about minerals. Like Dr Maurice Blackmore, I was concerned at Australia's ancient, depleted soils not adequately supplying our macro mineral needs. About ten years later I ran into a fellow student from the early 1990s, and he surprised me by saying "We all thought you were a bit mad with your talk about minerals and depleted soils. No one thinks that now". I suppose we need time to mull over ideas we have not thought about. One thing about Tasmania and a smaller population is that people more clearly can sort the wheat from the chaff. I was so lucky not to be considered a charlatan.

During this time at university I was still seeing patients and Juliet outgrew her pony. The next pony she chose was nearly as tall as a horse and looked like an Arab with fine legs, a ginger coat and thick golden mane and tail. She was a beauty and called Shanti. Like Toby, she had been put to grass for a couple of years and didn't want to be ridden, so lots of bucking and pig-rooting.

Again Juliet patiently re-trained her and rode her to pony club and she even won a first prize. A few years later, we sold Shanti but for some reason had to take her back and then she developed colic. It was over the Easter holidays and the vet was away. A riding friend of Juliet's called Susannah was staying with us. Both girls were aged 12,. They decided to nurse Shanti themselves. They brought her into the big open garage and gave her flat beer with a few magnesium phosphate tablets (65mgs) crushed into the beer. Of course they had difficulty getting the tablets into her. But they persevered at regular intervals and throughout the night. On the Sunday morning Susannah said to me "Mrs Fisher, I think Shanti is getting cold. She is shivering." So the girls added calcium phosphate tablets (65mgs) and continued the doses in flat beer for Sunday and much of the night. Next day Monday, finally the stomach of the horse was no longer a hard barrel and I was so proud of them for succeeding in nursing the poor animal through such a painful illness and back to good health. Looking back I think our soil was too poor for horses and should have had lots of limestone for better quality grass.

Before that, I think it was November 1992 when I came home one day on a Friday afternoon and there was no dog to greet me. I was in the middle of exams at the university. We had a Finnish girl living with us through the week. She and her father lived on Bruny Island but she stayed with us through the week so she did not to have to leave so early for school in Kingston. Friday night, neither my daughter nor Elinor (our Finnish girl) were there and I went out. Still no dog when I got back. In the morning Josephine the dog was in the kennel and could not get out so I took her to Barry Wells, our very popular vet. He thought it may be snake bite and put her on a drip. By Saturday afternoon he rang and said he was now sure it was snake bite and the antivenene was $200 which I did not have. Juliet brought down her Pat Colby horse book and found from it that Vitamin C was very useful in snake bite for horses. So I rang around and found a lady called Pat Woolley who had horses and gave one Vitamin C for beestings. This lovely person who lived in Margate brought a vial of Vitamin C to Barry Wells who asked if I was sure about injecting it into the dog's hind leg. The poor dog screamed but I took her home and she walked around the house and collapsed. Well I had two young girls living there so could not simply let the poor dog die without at least trying the minerals. So twice daily I powdered up the minerals I knew were needed to help the liver and kidneys to rid the body of the poison and to repair possible tissue damage and together with Vitamin C, honey or molasses in water managed to get the mixture down the dog's throat. During the day when we were at school and university I put the dog outside in semi-shade and brought her in at night. Barry Wells was wonderful. He rang each day and I told him about the pupils of the eyes changing, one almost filling the eye, the other a pinpoint, then opaque covers over the eyes. Barry explained about the breaking down of the central nervous system. Another vet, a woman also rang for daily reports and I told her I thought the dog would die. The dog became rigid with its teeth bared. It looked dead but it was not. So it got its twice daily dose of minerals. The treatment started late on Saturday. The dog, which loved to catch tiger snakes and we had huge ones, must have been bitten sometime on the Friday so the poison was in its system for at least 24 hours before the doses were started. Snake venom is supposed to be most potent in the spring and here we were in November. Through the week the dog was blind and rigid until the Thursday night when to our surprise, it started lolling its head around. Then I gave it some food well watered down with its minerals. On Saturday it was outside again. It had not shown signs of moving yet, but in the late afternoon I took it out a big meal. It got up on its hind legs which were shaking and ate it all up. Then it crawled on its belly right across the paddock and did an enormous poo. I had to carry the dog back. To all our surprise, the dog made a complete recovery with all its functions and movements intact.

Towards the mid nineties, patients were being referred to me by a man from the Huon called Kevin Corby. Each person had debilitating problems and quite different from every other. It was unnerving. I was still nervous and very concerned about accurate prescribing for everyone who came to me, so this recommendation from a stranger who had not been a patient himself was even more worrying. Who then was this Kevin Corby? Apart from telling me his name, the prospective patients were reticent about him and somewhat suspicious of me and my abilities, but they were often desperate and very fortunately for my peace of mind, they all did well.

One of those people was a woman who was very debilitated with severe depression and exhaustion.. She was another who needed the potassium phosphate as one of her required minerals. She was under a psychologist who she liked very much and felt very dependent on. The problem for her was that the CBT (cognitive behavioural therapy) her psychologist recommended made her feel worse than before she started. She was so exhausted to start with and was very suspicious of the minerals. However, I persuaded her to take the minerals for a month, 6 times daily and told her that as her energy improved, she would find she could do the exercises and gradually get the benefit her psychologist was aiming for. I learned later that her father had developed dementia which had made her afraid, as he had started with many of her present symptoms. She went on improving on the minerals and I hope she stuck to them over the years. One has to wonder about increasing dementia and its relationship to diminishing soil and food nutrients and then generations of people living from depleted soils.

Eventually I met Kevin Corby. He made an appointment and arrived one day. I saw him get out of his car in front of the French window of my office, look round with a doubtful expression as he came up to the front door. He was a frail little man of Irish descent and had a powerful intellect. We had a long, very interesting conversation. I learned that Kevin was a pharmacist and devout Roman Catholic with a vast knowledge of Catholicism and Biochemistry. He loved nothing better than religious discussions with priests of his church. He was quite fascinated with the improving health of people who came to his pharmacy who had got onto the minerals and we struck an accord, when I told him that I had come to believe that the healing power in our bodies came from a directive intelligence we were lucky to have working for us.

~ Seven ~

HUONVILLE AND NORTH HOBART PHARMACIES.

I finished my undergraduate degree and one day ran into one of my former psychology student friends who told me about a new Masters Degree in Education called Counselling and Development which she thought I would enjoy. So I enrolled and had a particularly enjoyable, challenging three years with Associative Professor Carey Denholm in charge. He was a man with a huge intellect whom we respected. He was something of a perfectionist, but we loved him for his great generosity of spirit. We were so lucky to have him. One day I asked him "If our development occurs according to how our genes interact with the environment, with so many injections children have today, can we expect a proportion of them to become attracted to injecting?" "I hope not", he said. Our children today are raised on drugs. My generation was not. I know this is a sacred cow, but I wonder if we may avoid fast escalating auto-immune diseases, if children were given fewer, but the most essential vaccinations and the rest stored in case of need.

We students worked well together, finding lots of information from the library and arguing about the different perspectives presented to us. I was very attracted to Carl Rogers' counselling technique. In my work, I was regularly impressed about how important it was to listen, or get people to open up, and it was sometimes at the very end of a consultation when the most valuable information for prescribing would emerge. Now I am appreciating Eric Erickson and his stages of development and what we are supposed to be doing at different stages of our lives. I am observing the stage of passing on learning to others from the years of my work, which I am doing a bit late in the piece, but I really thought by now someone else would have written about a history with the minerals. There are practitioners all over Australia using minerals, but I am writing about using them as a sole modality and perhaps others are using them in conjunction with other treatments and may not have realised their significance to life itself.

I had finally finished my Masters degree and within the week, Kevin Corby was on the phone and said he wanted me to work on his pharmacy floor. I told him I needed a holiday and I was not going to go down over the big mountain range to Huonville to work for him when I was so exhausted. Kevin was quite persuasive, so against my better judgment, I began to drive regularly to Huonville and magnificent as that mountain range is I do not like driving regularly over it in an icy winter.

It was quite an experience. The girls on the floor and the pharmacists did not know what to make of me. One of the girls openly laughed at the minerals. She was a girl with a happy, open personality and certainly not afraid of her opinions. Another girl, who I later found had the same birthday as me was wonderful at the till, which had me bluffed. She would quietly say to do this and that until I got my confidence. One day Vicki, the girl who laughed at the minerals got herself into distress. She was a party girl, who for some time had been drinking too much so she decided to take milk thistle to cleanse her liver. She became violently ill and stopped the tablets, but still felt quite nauseous. Finally she asked for help and I got her to take a tablet with magnesium phosphate and sodium sulphate, which she quickly responded to and stayed on for some time, while the liver symptoms vanished and she felt well. Then she became the greatest promoter of minerals in the pharmacy.

Kevin Corby used to say regularly "I know the minerals work, I just don't believe it, that's all!" I said to him "And don't you think that it may be a handful of minerals that God made us from? You can see how well they seem to restore our health". One day I was invited home for dinner by his wife June, a bubbly, busy person, quite a contrast to her aesthetic husband. She made me very welcome. Kevin showed me his paddocks where he grazed cattle. The top paddock was empty. He said DDT was used in the 1920s and even 70 years later, cattle still got sick and died if put in that paddock.

Kevin helped finance a new big pharmacy in Huonville. I had enjoyed some freedom until then. We were a very happy team who celebrated our birthdays over lunches, pharmacists and girls together and laughed and joked as we worked. I was paid the same as girls on the floor, about $12 an hour, but for me it was a learning experience. People came into the pharmacy to see me when they would not have paid for a consultation. I got to know all the products and occasionally recommended herbs. One young girl who had just started her periods broke out with bad skin and temper tantrums. I gave her Vitex Agnus Castus. By the next period she came in with her mother and there was hardly a bump on her skin "And best of all" said her mother "is that we can live with her. She's herself". The girl smiled and continued with the herb for some time. I later heard that monks in abbeys in Europe took Vitex Agnus Castus which supports progesterone production which helped to keep other hormone levels normal including testosterone. What a shame that we lose knowledge over time, with our modern ideas pushing out what may be old but true.

Kevin Corby had one each of herb tablets that Blackmores used to make. I had been working at the pharmacy for only a few days when a woman came in who had severe burning pain in her stomach, which she said was from taking Voltaren ® and the doctor had sent her to the pharmacy for help. I asked Kevin if the lady could have the harpagophythum (devil's claw) and hoped she'd get quick results. Next day she came and said the tablet had worked a miracle. Blackmores had a name for using the best product ingredients.

Another woman was taking a very high dose of thyroxine daily, which she said made her feel ill. She wanted to get off the thyroxine. I said that if the thyroid gland was functioning insufficiently she may not be able to do so. So she compromised and bought kelp tablets which showed the amount of iodine and she reduced the thyroxine gradually. She agreed to tell her doctor what she was doing. Over time she was able to maintain the thyroxine at a much lower dose, taking more of the kelp tablets. She was feeling well at last and agreed she may always need the smaller dose of the thyroxine she was now taking. There is no iodine in the soil in Southern Tasmania, or even in the rock dust in this part of the world, so lots of thyroid problems.

The new Huonville Pharmacy experienced some government interference and I fell out with a controlling person who did not appreciate someone not prepared to be just a cog in the wheel. Meanwhile I received an offer for an interview at Jerry Hampton's pharmacy in North Hobart Kevin Corby said "Don't go. Things will get back to normal" but I had already accepted the offer and I would not have so far to travel. Just the same, I missed those happy times with the girls and pharmacists in Huonville and they still sell both the minerals I introduced and the range of Active Elements ® I later came to use privately and in other pharmacies.

At this time in the 1990s, there was no natural health department in pharmacies in North Hobart. Jerry Hampton himself kept a tight ship and for the first year I often felt him over my shoulder seeming to listen to my advice to customers. He even built me a little consulting room. Again it was a happy place with lovely pharmacists but I heard that elsewhere a pharmacy paid the naturopath more. I helped the naturopath at this other pharmacy with mineral advice and she told me to apply for her job, when she went overseas.

Meanwhile life was busy in North Hobart, with all sorts of different advice sought. One day at the front counter I was talking to a couple from Sydney. They were on holiday but her debility was taking the edge off things. "I have heavy metal poisoning" she said "And I am disappointed that I am not up to climbing the Nut, Stanley where we are heading." I asked about her symptoms and gave her Blackmores Chloride and Sulphur compounds, (no longer produced.) I think I remember so well, because a short time later the couple again came into the pharmacy, this time to tell me she was very pleased, she had felt well enough to climb the Nut. "I felt better almost immediately and will stay on these tablets until I feel quite well". Usually heavy metal poisoning can take some time, but perhaps that depends on how much is stored in body tissues or is still mainly in the circulation.

One experience I cannot forget was about a young man whose wife came into North Hobart Pharmacy just after 5.00 p.m. one evening to ask the pharmacists for help with her husband, whose blood test that day showed abnormally high levels of phosphorus. I was called over. The young man was outside in the car and he was fetched in. He stood rigid against the wall of my consulting nook and I heard about how he could not sleep at night, was very depressed, yet felt he had no need to be and various symptoms that indicated to me that he was losing phosphorus from the cells into his bloodstream. Phosphorus is a very important anion in our metabolisms, directing the cations of potassium, magnesium, calcium, iron and sodium for specific structural purposes. His symptoms indicated the need for those cations which required the phosphorus anion, so I prescribed these low dose minerals, observing the cation/anion relationship, to be taken two hourly and during the night if he could not sleep. Next day or the day after he had another blood test which showed a normal phosphorus level. He stayed on the minerals for some weeks feeling better all the time.

Finally he said there was only one thing bothering him. At the end of each day he went into a panic attack. I asked him where he came from. "Bosnia", he said, and this was the 1990s. So I said I thought there was an experience from the war that was so horrific, he had suppressed it and this is where psychology can come into its own. I told him about my friend Robert who was also a hypnotherapist and had helped his beautiful wife who came from the Middle East who had experienced bombing and death of her class mates as a child. I suggested that if the frightening experience could be externalised, it would no longer bring on the panic attacks. I suggested we get in touch with the Migrant Resource Centre where he may be helped free of charge. He insisted on seeing Robert, who charged him half price. After 2 visits to Robert and hypnotherapy, he was free of the panic attacks. He stayed on the minerals a bit longer. Years later I met this couple and their children in the street and there had been no more problems. Robert used to go to a coffee shop in North Hobart where the wife of the young man worked. Thereafter Robert said he had free coffees.

One day one of the pharmacists at North Hobart Pharmacy recommended a big man to see me. He had been complaining about being unable to think or function well. He could not think properly and he blamed this on his drug medication for epilepsy. He was in his late forties and said he had taken Tegretol ® since the age of 7. His mother later told me that he was born an unusually big baby and they dropped him at birth and she wondered if the epilepsy was as a result of this. She was quite a small woman, so I imagine the birth must have been difficult.

He told me that he wanted to get back the clarity of thought he had experienced for a week following brain surgery in Melbourne 2 years earlier. He was a determined man who managed to work in his trade by writing down phone conversations and instructions immediately as he could not retain anything otherwise. He was taking two drugs, one of them being Tegretol® at 900 mg a day. He was still experiencing regular fitting despite the medications.

Gradually over months the fitting became minimal and he decided to take less of the Tegretol®. I told him to be very careful, as Tegretol® would be part of his normal biochemistry after taking it from his childhood. Very gradually he reduced the dose, experiencing a little more fitting, then taking a good break and allowing himself to adjust to the slightly lower dose, before again reducing the Tegretol® a little again. Over many months he was down to 200mg Tegretol®. He was thinking clearly, remembering things, and even having political arguments he never could do before. I wanted him to stop reducing the dose at this point, as I thought he had achieved a good balance with his health and didn't want to risk bringing on more fits again.

Then I did not see him for quite a while by which time I was working at Edwards Pharmacy. Apart from 3 mineral combinations 4 times daily, I had advised him to take Blackmores Plantiodine tablet once daily. He was a single man and although he had agreed on dietary improvements, I thought the Plantiodine, with its 1,000 mg Kelp, Rose hips, Brewers Yeast and Vitamin E would be a good supplement. He was a big man who I thought needed lots of good nutrition. He came back because he thought the minerals were no longer working. The confusion in his brain had returned. I couldn't understand it and got him to have a consultation with our head pharmacist. We could not work it out. Then I suddenly remembered the Plantiodine which Blackmores had discontinued 6 months earlier. "When did you have the last Plantiodine?" I asked. "Months ago", he replied. I went out to the shelves and took down a 1,000 mg kelp tablet container and told him to take one tablet twice daily with his minerals until his thinking processes became clear again. He rang me nearly two weeks later and said he was good again now. We reduced the kelp tablet to one a day and kept the mineral tablets at 4 times daily. He was a big man who needed regular amounts of the building block minerals. But it's very interesting to note that the trace element of iodine, when grossly lacking can throw out the balance attained by the macro minerals.

We are in a part of the world, where not only is iodine lacking in the soil, but even in the rocks that make crusher dust. To me this case demonstrates the interaction that occurs biochemically. I prefer that trace elements when added to the diet are in sea vegetables which supply so many tiny nutrients some of whose value may not yet be known.

I would like to say this was the end of the story. But he would not give up on trying to get off the Tegretol® and trying to force the pace. He also visited a chiropractor who stimulated the brain, which may have helped stir up the fits again. We had already been through him taking gingko blloba to stimulate his brain and the fits came on again and I said "no more stimulating the brain". Then he had a fit after a visit to the chiropractor and he was driving, and had a car accident and that was the end of his working life.

He seems to have finally accepted that he can't get off the Tegretol®l and I hope is having no more brain stimulation and sticking with the minerals that have supported him through all the experimentations. Although I wish he was not so stubborn, I applaud him for his courage. We learn from people like him, with the courage. to never give up.

An older woman asked me one if the minerals might help with her chronic sinusitis. She had reached the stage where the congestion seemed to have set like concrete. It was spring when it was at its worst and she said she was in agony. I told her that it may take many days for the congestion to move with the minerals as the sinusitis had been suppressed for so many years. I gave the minerals with the sulphur and potassium salts for cleansing with small amounts of silica to break up the congestion. She came to me a week later. "When is something going to happen? I am in such pain". I told her that I did not know, but if the was taking the small doses of minerals two hourly, I believed the stuck mucus would start to move. There days she came in and said she was losing tons of mucus and the pain had all but gone. She was jubilant. I was so relieved, but I did not know how else to help her.

On my last day at Jerry Hampton's pharmacy, a lady thanked me because the mineral supplement I had recommended to her in the week I arrived two years earlier worked for her and she now took her medication from the doctor without nausea or other problems. I had also been complemented by a local doctor for helping the health of people who were his patients. He said I seemed to be doing a good job, a quite unexpected compliment.

~ Eight ~

AT EDWARDS PHARMACY.

The years at Edwards Pharmacy led to me writing in magazines and a wonderful experience of working in a beautiful environment, the loveliest pharmacy I have ever seen. There was a beautician and child health nurse too. Kingborough was the fastest growing area in Tasmania and the pharmacy had been carefully designed to welcome a wide range of customers. It was comfortable for the pensioners and disabled and the locals regarded it as a regular meeting place and all of us, including the pharmacists made everyone welcome. Customers came up from the Huon where I had worked and the Huonville Pharmacy introduced the new mineral range I had introduced to Kingston. This was where I first became aware that pharmacists double-checked doctors' scripts to ensure that new medications would not cause problems with any other existing medications someone was already on.

By now I myself and customers who came to see me, regarded basic mineral therapy as their required treatment. It is amazing that simply addressing the minerals in their biochemical format respecting the cation/anion relationship would set into motion healing processes that led to restoration and maintenance of health with the only intervention being changes in formula if symptoms showed the need. It still amazes me after all these years, how Nature sorts out the order of healing. No matter what the health problem, so many of those that were considered medically recalcitrant would respond to the minerals and people came expecting this to happen, or occasionally to convince themselves that they had tried everything. It was still years before I realised that the principals I had learned applied in all of Nature which has led to my concern today about any lack of these elements and their availability due to increasing imbalances in our environment, particularly increasing atmospheric levels of carbon dioxide.

I had just started working at Edwards Pharmacy, when a desperate mother spoke to me about the sleeping problems of her son. I asked about his symptoms and prescribed potassium, magnesium phosphate with sodium sulphate (for his restlessness). I was sure he would sleep but next day his mother came in and told me he didn't. I told my boss who was surprised at my disappointment with myself. He said I would be lucky to get results 70 per cent of the time. However I always expected at least some results and told people that if I prescribed correctly, the results would come, to please let me know if this was not the case. I had learned by now, that the macro and trace minerals in the format our bodies were designed for are the elements of life and without them, even vitamins do not work well. They are our basic biochemistry for the functions of our metabolisms and it is better to use them in small, regular doses like we should be getting adequately in food and in the form created from our plant life, which converts the minerals into living food for us and all animal life.

One young Greek Australian lady came to see me one day. She was going through a bad divorce. I heard from a neighbour that her husband was violent and she was afraid. Her nerves were very bad and there were other problems. I had her back in two weeks. I was worried about her. Some symptoms had improved but she was still "a nervous wreck". I couldn't understand it. I went over the symptoms carefully and the minerals were right and then suddenly I noticed something I should have observed in the first place. One side of her face had dropped slightly. "Have you had Bells Palsy" I asked? "I am just getting over it". I gave her one more tablet, silica, which apart from breaking down arthritis helps heal nerve damage. She rang me a few days later and said she felt much better now with each day, so the silica was helping the potassium and magnesium phosphates in their work. for the nervous system.

A man came to see me who was in charge of road works that entailed a lot of very noisy drilling. He suffered from ringing in the ears that had become unbearable. His job therefore had become a nightmare. Fortunately he responded quickly on the minerals needed for what I considered to be nerve damage but he found that long term he needed to take regular small doses of the prescribed minerals so that he could continue with his job.

I saw a number of children at this pharmacy. I remember one little boy who had growth problems. He could not run, so missed out on sport and was expected to be operated on when he was a few years older. He took the minerals I thought he needed over the next few years, including calcium phosphate essential for bone growth and density. After about 10 years had gone by, there were new regulations in pharmacy and Edwards changed hands and soon the building too was destroyed and replaced by a carpark. I did not see this child again after that, but his mother rang me a few years later, when he was having sleeping problems and said his growth had become normal, he could now run, played sports and did not need the surgery.

Another little boy was diagnosed with ADHD and his parents did not want him on drugs so according to his symptoms, I prescribed two mineral compounds. I saw the parents from time to time and they said that as long as they kept him on the minerals he was fine. Growing children have particular needs for growth as well as maintenance.

One day a 23 year old girl was wheeled in to see me hoping I could help with badly swollen legs, particularly the left one. She was on methadone to control the pain. She said she had Chronic Regional Pain Syndrome with secondary nerve pains in the left leg. She was trying to retrain the brain, so she could walk a little. Her foot had been operated on from a bike accident when she was a child. She had developed an ulcer after the accident. Now her very swollen leg showed ulceration on the skin and looked fungal. Her skin dried, flaked and became "insanely" itchy and raw underneath. She was also on an anti-epileptic drug and Endep. She was on Nexium for gastric reflux and also took a multi-vitamin. Frequently her face and arms went red and burning and she felt the need for cold air. Her foot was red raw and swollen and could weep through bandages. She said she experienced pain and electrical buzzing (shocks and burning) and could not warm her leg on a cold day. It felt like ice water running along her leg. She had psoriasis on her scalp and felt better in fresh air. I prescribed two mineral compounds, one with the sulphur and potassium minerals for deep cleansing and one with magnesium and sodium phosphate to help the nerves and acidity. I saw her three weeks later and she said that even on the first day there was a change in the skin on the leg which felt better. Progress seemed slow over the next few months, but this was a very bad condition that had developed over years. At one point she was using anti-fungal cream on spots at the back of her neck and on her arms. The itching improved quickly, thank goodness. The psoriasis improved. She said her leg had improved and she could go back to sleep more easily now. I saw her for about a year. Later the pharmacy changed hands and I wished that the girl in the wheelchair had improved more. Occasionally I got a phone call for advice and then after a few years she made an appointment "to get her minerals sorted out" she said. I was no longer working in the pharmacy so she came to see me at home. To my great surprise, she got out of the car with a crutch and walked in, no wheelchair. Her leg was still a bit swollen, but nothing like it had been. She said she had never really got off the minerals, so I advised her to stay on the combination of sulphur/potassium cleansing formula and the other one for her nervous system that also looked after the ph balance. I sometimes see a photo from her on Facebook but I believe she would come to see me if she felt she needed to. It was so wonderful to work in pharmacies where such people could be open to treatment they otherwise might not have the opportunity to try. I really am very grateful to all the pharmacists I worked for who provided this service to their customers.

One day a man arrived for minerals for his wife. He said he had been sent. His wife had fallen from a gangplank walking ashore from a cruise ship and had been crushed between the ship and the wharf. I don't know how they managed to get her back to Hobart, but she was in excellent hands with the thoracic neurosurgeon caring for her. So I prescribed the calcium phosphate, sodium phosphate, magnesium phosphate, silica and calcium fluoride I thought would help to repair the many broken bones. Months later, the lady herself came to see me. She said the neurosurgeon had strapped her up and she took the minerals and the neurosurgeon was now very happy with how she had healed. She wanted to meet me and stay on the minerals a bit longer, just to consolidate what she had achieved. The cells of our bodies are constantly using minerals in their biochemical format for our daily activities, so it's good when one can ensure essential nutrients are regularly available when apart from daily activities, healing also is needed.

Another lady with a long treatment period was one who was on Tamoxifan since 1989 following ovarian cancer. I saw her in 2004. She had brittle nails, sore neck, cold hands and feet and felt like a wave was moving from her eyes around her head and sometimes she felt like not eating at all. She was very concerned about losing her hair, which the skin specialist told her would not regrow. She was prone to oily skin and hot sweats and had sinusitis in the spring, could not sit still and could not stand heat and humidity. She stayed on the minerals, which I adjusted as needed and after a year, to her delight, her eyebrows grew back. She wore a lovely wig. "But what about my hair?" Two months later her hair began to grow back and she grew a lovely thick head of wavy hair. She said she would write to the skin specialist and tell him not to tell anyone again that their hair won't grow back after cancer treatment. I had told her that the hair follicles, being attached to the outer organ, the skin, would probably not respond to the minerals until her other internal health problems were resolved (Nature choosing the order of healing) and that's what happened.

One of my bosses from Edwards Pharmacy met me for coffee (this was after the pharmacy had been sold) and asked me if I remembered a man who had been in prison many times and took the minerals to try to stabilise his violent temper. He said he had met the man at church and the man told him that the minerals I had prescribed from his pharmacy had changed his life. In fact he changed his own life, by being prepared to help himself. I remembered how years earlier I had suggested to a Health Department person, that Blackmore's Magnesium compound (no longer produced) should be trialled in the prison system. Of course this did not happen.

Very occasionally I recommended a herb, despite preferring the elements of regeneration. One day a tall older man with very fragile skin arrived when I was standing at the ointments shelf. He had varicose eczema on his shins which he said nothing would help. I took down a jar of comfrey ointment and told him to rub it in several times a day. He came back a few weeks later and showed me his legs, where the skin had been weeping and open and now there was not a mark to be seen. This old pensioner was delighted. Yet it said on the jar not to use comfrey if the skin was broken. As comfrey is rich in calcium which repairs tissue and bones, I thought it would repair the skin and it did. One thinks about the actions that medicines, minerals, herbs etc. do and learns to consider one's judgment and decide accordingly.

I wonder why Vitex Agnus Castus was given up by Monks in monasteries! Vitex Agnus Cactus (chaste tree) was apparently taken by the Monks because it helped with celibacy. It is a herb which favours progesterone production that is required by both men and women. Progesterone acts powerfully and helps maintain hormonal balance.

One day I was reading a herb book in the pharmacy. There was a section about kelp and other sea vegetables and how they inhibited the uptake of iron in the gut. Australian soils are often rich in iron but lacking in iodine. So is hemochromotosis an imbalance where too much iron is absorbed when not regulated by other trace elements like iodine? At any rate, from thereon I advised people who said they had hemochromotosis to take kelp, which provided Nature's trace element formula in food form and hoped this simple action might help control some of the excessive iron.

A new medical centre was built to house the many G.Ps in the Kingston area and our pharmacy had an adjoining pharmacy built next to and part of the complex. One morning, one of my employers, Philipa Maxwell asked me for a few minutes and told me that the previous evening she had had a meeting with the doctors in the new complex and asked them how they felt about me and a few of them said they were quite happy about my services. But one of them said she had been standing near me one day in my department when I was asked a question about vaccination and she heard me say about how in Japan, children had not been vaccinated until the age of 2 because their immune systems were not considered mature enough until them (It may well be different now, but I think that was the case at the time).

That was the only other observation offered at the meeting. It was good to get a report on my value to the pharmacy and it reminded me of the importance of all of us working together for the good of the whole community.

At this time it was decided that the pharmacy needed a new carpet. Edwards Pharmacy was always full of people. As free tea and coffee was also provided and the open layout and beautiful decor in each department was inviting, their good quality carpet had become a bit worn. One of the carpet layers came to see me a week before the new carpet was to be laid. He said "I can't do the job with my right hand so swollen". It was twice the size of the left hand, a stress related problem from years of carpet laying. What to do! A new joint cream had arrived, glucosamine with capsicum. I told the man to rub the cream into his hand as often as possible over the next week. He and a mate arrived a week later to lay the new carpet. He showed me his hand, which had returned to normal size. He said he could still feel it but could do the job. I saw him again about two years later. He came to tell me a story about climbing down to a waterfall in a national park, which years earlier he could not do, because of his damaged knees from carpet laying and that he was due to have surgery for. He said he had beaten his wife down to the waterfall. He said that since he had last visited the pharmacy he had rubbed the glucosamine/capsicum cream into his knees three times daily without fail and his doctor had cancelled his knee replacements. As we know glucosamine is a joint food and capsicum is anti-inflammatory, but the minerals in the capsicum would no doubt have helped the absorption of the cream into his joints. I have told this man's story many times when recommending this cream.

One tiny woman who came to see me had had cancer of the oesophagus two years earlier and radio and chemotherapy. Now each morning she brought up stringy material and she also had bad sinusitis. I prescribed half doses of silica and a combination tablet with sulphur salts, i.e. potassium chloride, potassium sulphate, calcium sulphate, magnesium phosphate. I thought she needed the two half tablets 4 times daily, but because she was on Atacand Plus® for high blood pressure (an ace inhibitor that interferes with potassium absorption), I told her to take them to her doctor and we would refund her money if she was not to take them. Apparently her doctor said the combination potassium, sulphur compound was miraculous. Others of his patients had taken this tablet. He told her that her blood pressure would go up for a week, then stabilise. Within a few months her sinusitis had gone and so had the stringy material she had been bringing up for two years. She now seemed quite well.

We had a hairdressing salon and one of the hairdressers was trying to get off antidepressants, but when she got to the lowest dose, the depression overtook her again. The problem was resolved with one tablet of potassium/magnesium phosphate with sodium sulphate (low dose) two hourly, but she had to take it at that dose for two weeks before gradually lowering it until the depression no longer occurred.

I have had very little experience in treating people with epilepsy but a quite beautiful gypsy looking mother brought along her little girl one day and asked if I could help with her epilepsy. I worked out from her symptoms what might help the child and the fitting settled down. I explained to them that the child's growth would also take the minerals, so she may need to stay on them until she reached puberty. At regular intervals after this, the mother would arrive, sent by her daughter who insisted the minerals really helped her.

While working at Edwards Pharmacy, I had three quite similar cases of early teenage girls who had years of bowel and digestive problems. They had also experienced their father leaving the family to make another life. No doubt they held their heartbreak tight in their stomachs. One girl had had enemas but still was suffering from bowel congestion. These are almost the only times I have recommended a mineral that was not in the bio-chemical format. The girls took magnesium oxide which if prop-erly done, will flush out the bowel with water, starting with the upper intestine to unblock it. Then the girls stayed on the min-erals in biochemical form to help their nervous systems and re-establish good bowel motions. One day one of the fathers visited me and told me the problem with his daughter was because of a teacher. I said "No it wasn't. It was because of you leaving home". It's a shame that it's unfashionable to sort out problems, rather than breaking things up. It would be much better for chil-dren to see that problems between people can reach a truce or even be resolved.

Another girl I worked with had a son who had broken a bone in his foot a few months earlier which was not mending. Only when time was running out before prospective surgery did she tell me about it. She hadn't mentioned it because her son was on warfarin. I assured her the tablet he needed would not interfere with the warfarin. As I remember, he had two weeks to go before an X-ray and possible surgery. So he took calcium phosphate, silica with calcium fluoride (homeopathic dose) twice daily. On the morning of the X-ray this mother was a nervous wreck but at lunchtime a joyous mother told me the X-ray showed budding of the bone to knit. When her son told his doctor what he was taking, the doctor apparently said he didn't care what he was taking but to stay on it. This combination of minerals provides the impetus of budding of new bone growth to knit.

I was reading in one of the herb books we had in the pharmacy about how sea vegetables like kelp inhibit the uptake of iron in the gut. I was seeing a number of people who had hemochromatosis. Iron is prevalent in rocks over 600 million years old and Australia is geologically ancient and the world's largest exporter of iron ore. So if soils are lacking iodine, but rich in iron, perhaps an imbalance regarding our metabolisms occurs. Today we are losing the rich kelp fields along the east coast of Tasmania, thought to be because of global warming, as sea water temperature has risen dramatically. So perhaps a general lack of iodine in our soils and diet leads not only to thyroid problems, but to hemochromatosis. Those most at risk are often Northern Europeans, who came from geologically much younger soils, so it may be that here in Australia, with our European ancestors, we over generations may be accumulating iron if iodine is severely lacking in the diet. It's worth investigating.

One day I was glancing through the paper left on a table where customers sat while waiting for their prescriptions. There was an article from Kidney Australia about Australia's escalating kidney problems and anticipating a lack of dialysis machines to cope with growing needs. I had just seen a man who had reported on his latest kidney test which showed now normal kidney enzymes. He had visited me a month earlier with raised kidney enzymes.

Sodium sulphate helps the kidneys to balance fluid levels and to excrete heavy metals. Australia lacks sulphur in the soil, not surprising when there has been no volcanic activity for so many millions of years. Magnesium phosphate in small doses works well with sodium sulphate to help regulate kidney activity. I was becoming increasingly frustrated at how ignorant we are about our requirements for minerals from our soils. Yet there have been previous generations of children who were raised on sulphur and treacle. So I rang Kidney Australia and spoke to the CEO in Adelaide and suggested that increasing kidney disease may primarily relate to sulphur deficiency in our soil, otherwise how could a simple sulphur mineral tablet on an average 3 times daily dose, help restore kidney enzyme level to normal within a very short time.

A young student who worked with us part-time, had a 30 year old horse with a hoof which had been swollen for months. The vet had not been able to help. The problem was resolved within 10 days with 65mg potassium chloride tablets, 5 tablets twice daily. I had learned that all species need the same biochemistry for the same purpose.

Recently I met with one of my employers from Edwards Pharmacy and we had coffee together. He told me about a man who now goes regularly to his church who had recently told him how the minerals had changed his life. He had been in and out of jail for years when he was violent and unstable. He said he would always stick to the minerals I had put him on, as now he was happy and working in a regular job.

I remembered how some years earlier there was a newspaper article about the violent behaviour of prisoners in jail. I wrote to the minister and told her about a magnesium combination from Blackmore's Laboratories, that I thought would make a difference and why not have a double-blind trial using this compound and a placebo. It's a shame that my suggestion came to nothing. On later learning from Europe that according to the International Fruiters Association, Cambridge, (more about this later), today's generation have 1/3rd the dietary intake of potassium of previous generations. The mineral compound had (it's been discontinued) a small amount of potassium phosphate, very helpful when people are miserable. If magnesium phosphate levels are also low, it's no wonder that one in four people today in the U.K. are depressed.

Over the years I worked in Edwards Pharmacy, I met many European new Australians. It seemed to become a recurring theme, that for some years (often about 7 years), the good health they had arrived with had remained, then they gradually developed health problems. If it was gluten intolerance, they found on return visits to Europe that they could eat foods with gluten as they had done previously, with no intolerance occurring. I explained that the cultivar of wheat that grows in Australia seems to be very high in gluten, so it might be better to avoid Australian products that are high in gluten like wheat.

It seemed like common sense to me to encourage people to eat according to their genetic predispositions, Asians continuing to eat rice in preference to wheat etc. I usually asked about people's inherited diets and suggested their health might benefit better from what had become familiar over many generations.

I worked at the beautiful and happy Edwards Pharmacy for over 10 years. By the end of this time, after seeing perhaps thousands of people, I found it difficult to understand why modern medicine did not give significance to the cellular foundations of our biochemistry and also why there was such fear about how Nature may treat us. We shall never win battles with Nature, but helping Nature with elements used in repair and cleansing does work. After all, in building construction, the foundations are crucially important. The minerals are foundational to our biochemistry, so aren't they just as crucial as the foundations of a building structure?

~ Nine ~

ABC TV SECOND OPINION.

About halfway through 2005 I received a telephone call from ABC Television, Hobart. Would I like to participate in Second Opinion, a program that was already running. They would like me to provide two different patients for two appointments each, six weeks apart. They would film the appointments and also interview myself and the patients separately. Due to time pressures, the first interviews were hastily put together and I asked two of my new patients if they would be happy to appear on television. They were both interested and their problems were quite different.

The first patient was a lovely young woman from the Huon. She desperately wanted to lose weight. Her main problem was that she always felt hungry. It is quite common for people to become overweight because they never feel satisfied. Such people can eat a meal at night and then raid the cupboard, but no matter how much they eat, they do not feel satisfied. I believe it's potassium phosphate they are craving, because within the first two weeks the appetite becomes normal. I say to such people, don't hate yourself. Your appetite is driving you to find an essential mineral compound, your body is desperately craving.

This lady knew about minerals used in agriculture and told me that down the Huon, potassium was used in the soil for the cherry orchards. The soil was checked each year for the nutrients needed for a good crop of cherries and potassium was regularly applied This did not surprise me as I had learned a valuable lesson from a university lecturer in agronomy about lack of potassium in the soil in this part of the world.

One day a professor of Agriculture came into my health department at Edwards Pharmacy. I was mulling over so many people's apparent need for additional potassium. I said to him "Why am I always finding that people require potassium in one form or another?"

He said, "I can't tell you about people. I can only tell you about soils."

"Please tell me then."

"The underlying soil structure in Southern Tasmania is dolorite. Potassium goes straight through it. It does not stay in the soil."

A lightening bulb flashed in my mind. I remembered the organic gardener who told me he could not keep potassium in his soil and if many people were of Irish descent, they were not being helped either, living in a part of the world where potassium does not stay in the soil and neither were the rest of us for that matter.

This lady with whom I discussed lack of potassium and how the specific need for potassium phosphate often drove people to eat in excess, was weighed at her first appointment and six weeks later at her second appointment with Tasmanian ABC TV. The difference in weight was remarkable. Not only had she lost a very noticeable amount of weight, but she was a very pretty woman and at this second viewing, she glowed with health.

My second patient was a two year old boy who was severely autistic. His mother had come to me as a patient herself while her husband carried this beautiful child with vivid blue eyes and thick dark hair, over his shoulder as he walked round the pharmacy waiting for her. I noticed that the eyes of the little boy did not seem to focus on anything going on around him. I was just finishing with his mother when she asked if I could help this child. So I asked what he would eat (thinking how to get the minerals into him). "You can never tell. Sometimes he seems to like something and the next day will spit it out". So I gave her a sample of a powder for children that made into a drink sweetened with sucralose and contained most of the building block minerals and I said a prayer that he would like it.

At the same time as I first saw the mother and child, the ABC rang me and the mother was quite happy for her little boy to be part of the program. The child was filmed at home in a lifeless and unhappy state, not registering a full nappy and often screaming all night and not even relating to his parents or older brothers.

On the second visit of the ABC cameramen to the family home six weeks later, a very different picture was filmed. I heard about it when the cameramen arrived at the pharmacy. To my surprise, one of them apologised to me. "We thought you were a charlatan. That little boy was like a vegetable when we first saw him. Today he was sitting on the floor doing a puzzle. We couldn't believe the change in him."

I was very glad that he had only been severely autistic for about 6 months, so responded quickly. He was developing naturally, the same as his brothers and became suddenly autistic. Over the years we had observed how children's mental and emotional abilities can change quickly on the minerals. I had added a small dose of silica powdered in the drink which contained the phosphates for growth, potassium, magnesium, calcium and sodium for the pH balance. Later he was on three mineral compounds (much cheaper for the parents) : one of which was potassium and magnesium phosphate, calcium and sodium phosphate and silica with homeopathic fluoride. Later he took the minerals twice daily but more often if there was a growth spurt.

When this little boy (Ruben) was five I wrote an article about him in Tasmanian Life magazine, December 2009/January, 2010, a lovely Christmas story. There were photographs of him writing his name and jumping on the trampoline. He was now able to share a room with one of his brothers. I asked him as we were leaving if I could give him a kiss on his cheek. He said "Of course." As I left he called out "Goodbye." He seemed to have become a normal happy little boy.

Today he would like to become an architect but his family has hit hard times. His wonderful mother had a bad car accident, can't work and is living on Newstart while waiting for surgery and the child at adolescence could do with the help of minerals which he has not had for some years now. He is also good at gymnastics and I think is already a person who will achieve in life against all the odds.

In the 1970s when we saw so many children, I used to think that every child would benefit from potassium/magnesium phosphate and calcium/sodium phosphate which were the minerals Ruben took finally. I remember a teacher in Kingston asking me "How can you teach children with a 5 minute attention span?" Those particular minerals essential for growth may well be the answer. Certainly they are in my experience. The situation seems much worse today than when I was a child. We were usually in classes of 60 or more and we learned. We had an exam at the end of each year and mostly passed into the next year. There was a standard we seemed capable of meeting, but of course our soils had double the mineral level (Dr Marten Stapper, CSIRO agronomist, 1/6/2009) and we had stale sandwiches on Mondays - no preservatives. If the minerals increase children's concentration and attention span as I've so often witnessed, we must expect a learning deficit when essential minerals are below levels necessary for optimum development.

I was told by one of the ABC people, that my episodes on Second Opinion where I was questioned about the minerals, brought in hundreds of phone calls. One of the callers managed to find me at home. He was a supplier of minerals to farmers in Western Australia. He thanked me because he was suddenly inundated with requests from farmers for minerals for their crops. He said it had been hard to get the farmers to buy minerals for their soils and now there was suddenly a big demand for the minerals. I think it is wonderful that when farmers realise that our health depends on the minerals their plants provide, they will spend hard earned money to build up their soils.

One day I was listening to the noonday Saturday Science Show on Radio National. A volcano had just gone off in New Zealand and a vulcanologist from New Zealand was asked about it. It was the last thing he said that really interested me. He said that there was not much lava, "not enough for my garden, worse luck". It was obvious that he knew that the volcanos spewed out minerals which enrich our soils.

We in Australia are without this natural refertilisation of the soil, but we might do a deal with Indonesia where I believe there is a volcano which bubbles along at ground level and is wasted for them, as their soils receive fairly regular volcanic fallout in their rains. Perhaps northern Australia gets a little Indonesian volcanic fallout in the summer cyclones. At least we should think about this and how we can better help our farmers, particularly in central and southern Australia.

England during the years of World War 2 until the mid 1950s demonstrated what can happen with a nation's health when people are living almost exclusively from limestone rich soil, despite terror and destruction to homes from often daily bombings. Growing children have a particular need for calcium phosphate which makes our bones and children growing up at this time in England grew a head taller than their parents, despite the deprivations. People were under-nourished in calories, children were skinny, but they were healthy despite the chaos of war, families separated, particularly children separated from parents to protect them from city bombings, U.S. military vehicles sometimes driving on the wrong side of the road and regular destruction to people and infrastructure. By the time I moved to England, rationing had been discontinued for some years, and I met families where cakes and sugary foods were now part of daily life. They were making up for years of deprivation without realising the increasing damage to their health. Like ourselves many British people today live on rubbishy take-away foods and like us there is an escalating health bill

~ Ten ~

TASMANIAN LIFE MAGAZINE.

In 1997 I was asked to write for Scene magazine which was a free community magazine for Kingborough and the Huon. I wrote articles for a few editions of Scene magazines.

This led to me being asked to write for Tasmanian Life, a beautiful glossy magazine found in doctors' waiting rooms and hotel rooms and lobbies, apart from on magazine stands. It cost $11.95 to start with and it came out seasonally. I was always looking for interesting themes for my articles and the ABC Health Report was one program which gave me inspiration and the chance to research and provide another opinion to their health programs.

One of the earlier articles I wrote in Tasmanian Life was about dementia, which by 2010 when I wrote my article had become newsworthy. In my article I wrote about Dr Gregory Cole, PhD, Professor of Medicine and Neurology at UCLA David Geffen School of Medicine and Associate Director of Geriatric Research Education who noted, that autopsies revealed that in the brains of aged Asians from India, the brains were stained yellow from their dietary curry, but had significantly youthful cell densities in the cortex of their brains, unlike approximately half the amount in the brains of British people the same age. Curcumin in turmeric, integral to curries is rich in nutrients like iron, vitamin B6, potassium and manganese. Churchmen (Science 2004) proved to benefit people with cystic fibrosis. It seems likely it's rich in potassium chloride because the thick mucus that builds with cystic fibrosis is corrected. It clears inflammation and pain and crosses the blood brain barrier, so may help clear detritus that can later be found as dementia develops. Two thirds of dementia sufferers live in the developed world. When I wrote this article, 2.6% of India's population had dementia. In Australia it is expected that 25% of the population will get dementia. To me these differences say plenty about processed, refined food as well as soil deficiencies. Every year in India, the monsoons wash down nutrients from the geologically younger Himalayas and replenish India's soils enriching largely vegetarian diets. In Australia our soil is ancient and we are far away from volcanic fallout and earthquakes that might bring to the surface minerals from deep within. Nor do we have geologically younger mountains to wash nutrients down from.

In another article in 2010 I wrote about The Case for Calcium Phosphate. I took my inspiration for this article from a "landmark" study reported by Dr Norman Swan on the ABC Health Report, who said that these results have not been replicated. The trial was reported in the April 1994 edition of the British Medical Journal. It was called "Effect of Calcium and Cholecalciferol treatment for three years on hip fractures in elderly women." The women took a daily dose of 1.2 grams of calcium and 800 i.u. cholecalciferol over 18 months. The trial was conducted in France with 3270 mobile elderly women around 84 years of age from 180 nursing homes, with half the women on the active tablets ingredients and half on a double placebo. The results were highly significant and also showed a continued preventive effect of calcium phosphate with cholecalciferol. An annual injection of calciferol was suggested, but this by itself did not significantly reduce the number of hip fractures. An Australian study using a "loading" dose of vitamin D (because it stores in the body at the beginning of winter) on 2,256 women actually showed a 26% INCREASE in fractures and falls, the highest incidence occurring in the first three months. I wondered how it was expected that people lacking vitamin D could be successfully forced to absorb a "loading" dose. It seemed counter intuitive to me.

I wondered what form of calcium was used in the highly successful French study and found it was tri calcium phosphate, the same as in the tablets I prescribe myself. The form of mineral supplementation and the balance is important, remembering that how we absorb is decided by nature. Phosphate is an anion and superphosphate used in agriculture is very powerful, yet cations like calcium used with it are lower in Australia than in many other countries, yet our soils may need even greater amounts of calcium, magnesium, potassium, sodium (cations) with the (anion) phosphate to address soil imbalances, or we may expect imbalance to our grasses and other food plants. Calcifications in soft tissue, believed to result from taking calcium tablets, raises the question of form. It's needed as a phosphate for bone and circulation and silica breaks down calcifications. Silica is known as the calcium organiser.

From Les Fisher's seminars in England during the 1980s, the medical doctor with the largest homeopathic practice in England had changed his practice over to mineral therapy. In February 1984, the Herald Sun published an article taken from the Observer in London. It was titled "Arthritis : The Mineral Alternative". The story was about a 73 year old nursing sister who was bedridden waiting for a double hip replacement operation. She could not get to see Dr Sherwin who sent the minerals to her, also diagnosed by hair analysis. "Before I started taking the tablets I could not move a leg". Dr Sherwin advised about diet and exercise too. They did not meet until she could walk 18 months later. She said she had seen both sides of medicine and wrote to Prince Charles and the Observer newspaper and The Herald/Sun picked up the article and published it.

Calcium phosphate is the largest mineral compound in the human body providing bone and maintenance of good circulation. Growing children have a great need, so living in a country where calcium producing rock like limestone is scarce becomes very challenging for producing good bone structure and when calcium combines with fluoride (also in short supply), if both these minerals are lacking, we can expect all sorts of connective tissue problems, apart from the enamel of our teeth. The Health Department when deciding on fluoride in the water supply might have done better to check with basic biochemistry. They would have found that what we needed fluoride as calcium fluoride.

As I am writing a memoir, it may be appropriate to tell my own calcium story. My mother was one of those who were close to starving during he Great Depression of the 1930s. I was her first child, born in 1941 and she was very anaemic and I realise now was also calcium deficient I was born quite different structurally from the rest of the family. I grew into a child who was badly knock kneed, flat footed, hair so thin you could see the scalp and badly chewed nails. I can remember picking up pencils with my toes. I don't remember the callipers which did not work anyway. At the age of 7 my mother decided I should be operated on by Dr Meehan, Australia's top orthopaedic surgeon at the time. She'd heard of Dr Maurice Blackmore who was practising in Brisbane then. "He looks in your eyes, ha, ha, ha," I can still remember her saying. I so needed the calcium phosphate I am sure he would have given me. But I went to the Mater Hospital. I can remember leading the prayers at 5.00 p.m. They were very generous because I was not a Catholic. I had bones broken and moved and was in plaster up to my chest while the bones healed. That was August. At Christmas I walked with my parents and brother between Lake Eacham and Lake Barrine on the Atherton Tableland - 14 miles. We were camped at Lake Eacham where I learned to swim.

I was just over 70 when my hips collapsed together and I had hip replacements. There was a lot of arthritis and now I have my knock knees back. Of course I am now taking the requisite minerals but in my case, with collapsed hips, I could not have stayed in bed for 18 months, but it seems to me that great pressure was put on the hip joints over the years, with my bones put into other positions than they were growing in. I've danced in cabaret in London which I could not have done with knock knees. I've carried my pack over the South Coast track and Overland track here in Tasmania and I accept that originally the surgeon did his best for me, but I can't help thinking "If only my mother had taken me to see Maurice Blackmore". It makes me feel grateful and humble that I've seen over time, how minerals have corrected abnormal bone growth in children.

Another article I wrote in a 2010 edition of Tasmanian Life was about Lifestyle & Stress and potassium and magnesium phosphates were key minerals I wrote about. At the time, magnesium was being given in New Zealand jails to see if it had a calming effect on prisoners. If it was given in the form of magnesium phosphate I am sure it would have been found to be beneficial.

I had been given a paper sent to the Department of Agriculture, UTAS from Cambridge, U.K. This paper called "Beneficial Effects of Potassium on Human Health" had been presented by The International Fertiliser Society in May 2007. It stated that in most developed countries, people today consume ONE THIRD the amount of potassium than previous generations, which they attributed to processed foods and people eating less fruit and vegetables. Soil deficiencies, or factors inhibiting plant uptake of potassium was not mentioned. The article spelled out proven medical requirements of potassium for heart and blood pressure. Renal disease may also be slowed or prevented by increased potassium in the diet. The article pointed out that potassium is regarded as the most important intracellular cation in the human body.

I pointed out in my article that potassium works according to the action of the anion (negative charge) and with phosphate therefore is most often restorative in mental and emotional situations. I have seen it often quickly successful in cases of extreme grief as well as exhaustion. It is essential for growing children to help their physical and mental energy and memory and concentration and sense of wellbeing. Whereas for glandular problems, where there is swelling, white pus and/or white mucus, it is potassium chloride the metabolism is calling for, not in the medical 500 mg dose, but often regular 2 hourly doses of 50 mg. It heals ulcerative conditions. Often glandular fever requiring potassium chloride and/or other minerals is followed by chronic fatigue, when the metabolism is becoming exhausted and potassium phosphate may be needed to kick start and build up depleted energy. Potassium sulphate however, is often characterised by the need for fresh air, a problem when one is also lacking calcium phosphate, when the need for fresh air makes one feel colder. Potassium sulphate is needed for deep seated infections, usually successful with psoriasis and chronic sinusitis and helps control burning fevers that peak at the end of the day. It often helps with the burning heat of menopause.

In 2012 another article I wrote for Tasmanian Life I took from The New Scientist, November 2002 when they published an article called Plague of Plenty which examined research up to that time which found that as trees grow faster from absorption of increased atmospheric CO_2, nutrient intake declines.

At the same time as my article came out in Tasmanian Life's autumn 2012 edition, I saw an ABC TV Catalyst program called "Tree Deaths." The program was about trees all over the world, dying en masse in climatic conditions of extreme heat and drought. They showed a whole mountainside of dead trees in Switzerland, trees in Yosemite National Park and in South America, trees that two weeks earlier had seemed alive. I was so depressed I nearly turned the program off, but right at the end, scientists went out in extreme heat from Murdoch University in West Australia to huge gum trees splayed out dead on the ground and being eaten by worms. They gave the trees a plug of fungicide, then a plug of nitrogen, potassium, phosphate and trace elements. Within two weeks the "dead" trees were sprouting new twigs and leaves, coming back to life. I danced round the room. It tickled me that trees responded just like humans. I rang up and spoke to one of the scientists and told him that potassium phosphate is what I give my half-dead patients and they come back to life, often quickly too. I told him about the article I had in the current Tasmanian Life magazine and how I had read about the effect of atmospheric carbon dioxide on trees in the New Scientist in November, 2002.

This Catalyst program, Tree Deaths had a real impact on me which I found hard to understand. After all I had treated animals, horses, cats and dogs with the minerals as symptoms dictated, but essentially the same as for humans, so why shouldn't plants respond like other living creatures? For me, this was a landmark program uniting all of life in a specificity of mineral absorption for particular purposes. And how is it that medications, mineral or other go straight to where they are needed? There must be an intelligence which tries to promote life and which I hope we will not continue to undermine, thinking we know better than Nature. We are products, not creators of Nature.

But what also stood out to me was the understanding these agricultural scientists seemed to have about the cation/anion relationship of how the minerals work in living things. Sometimes I've found that older people can display many symptoms of lack of potassium phosphate, light headedness, lack of energy, particularly on waking, trouble with memory and concentration, general debility etc. yet a blood test shows normal potassium levels. Why then are there quite specific symptoms for potassium phosphate, or sometimes potassium chloride or potassium suilphate? I say to my patients, "you don't get symptoms for nothing" and in prescribing for the symptoms, irrespective of the blood level, the symptoms disappear and the blood levels remain normal. Then again, blood is the home of iron phosphate. Perhaps the blood circulation does not necessarily tell one what is happening at a cellular level in the organs of the body.

If the minerals of life cannot be destroyed and are needed for life's purposes in all species, then this does appear to indicate a basic law of nature applying to all of life. Dr William Schussler, who together with other doctors in the mid to late 1800s, discovered function and symptoms of requirements for these indestructible minerals, which he named Biochemistry. Schussler's Biochemistry was based on the macro minerals found in ash even after all other living matter was obliterated, and how a positive charged mineral combines with a negative charged mineral for specific functions. And the minerals in life do not die. They can be active in life again after all else has decayed or been incinerated. It is wonderful to think that we can neither create nor destroy the minerals of life. We know they are found in volcanoes and on other planets. Silica and magnesium were found on Pluto, both essential for functions within our bodies. We should be particularly grateful to these doctors for working out the specific symptoms as they apply to mineral compounds. One can tell about symptoms from the tongue, iris, skin etc. but the most valuable thing of all for accurate prescribing is provided by a whole range of symptoms, experienced and particular to the individual person.

Referring back to The Effects of Carbon Dioxide becoming more and more excessive in the atmosphere, it eventually dawned on me that trees may be weakening with absorption of less minerals and protein and filling up with more cellulose, which may make them more vulnerable to weather extremes. Or is it the weather extremes altering moisture content that makes minerals more difficult to absorb? Nature seems to be using trees and our oceans to act as carbon sinks, but we are not sufficiently facing the fact that the increasing carbon dioxide may be leading in the direction of our destruction and the eventual destruction of all life as we know it, through increasing malnutrition.

Yet when carbon is used where soils have lost two thirds of their carbon content, improvement of soil and plants occurs. So I ask the question, do life's elements require various natural processes, particularly photosynthesis for plants themselves and animals to ultimately derive their nourishment? How much CO_2 in soils provides the best balance with other nutrients plants require for optimum health?

Another question I have is about the fluoride, which I believe is a residue from the aluminium industry and put into our water supply. Where calcium is adequate in the soil, we may have calcium fluoride which is required by all the connective tissue in our bodies ; skin, capillaries, ligaments, joints, etc. But what is the action of a forceful anion like fluoride when the cation of calcium is lacking? What about increasing skin cancers, aneurisms, joint and ligament weaknesses, etc.?

All life forms have been found to require less than three dozen elements. Therefore the lack of a single element puts great strain on living functions as the powerful life force tries to compensate, if one or more element becomes less available. These principles are laid down in the new science of Ecological Stoichiometry (Sterner and Eiser, 2002).

According to "Plague of Plenty", New Scientist, 2002, Hidden Hunger (micronutrient malnutrition) is the world's leading health problem. On 1/6/2009 Dr Marten Stapper, former CSIRO farming systems agronomist wrote in Soil Fertility Management, we need a balance of minerals and microbes for soil and human health. Over the past 60 years, mineral density in foods has declined to less than half of former levels. Practising mineral therapists observe symptoms of essential element deficiencies in almost everyone. Growing atmospheric CO_2 and/or global warming therefore is bad news for all of life and as Dr Maurice Blackmore explained to me, Australian soils may be worst off of all.

In 2012 I also wrote about Pesticides and Vitamin D. I had written in a 2009 edition of Tasmanian Life about toxins in Tasmanian soils following research by the Tasmanian government into ground water and bore water following excessive winter rain after a decade of drought. Underground water supplies had dwindled and were at a record low level in the Coal River Valley, Margate and Huon and were found heavily contaminated with chemicals. The herbicide atrazine was at 0.1 parts per billion. Atrazine was banned in Europe at 0.01 parts per billion.

In relation to vitamin D, joint US-Korean research J-H Yang et al, (Plos One, 2012,7) had found that pesticides may be suppressing vitamin D levels. They checked for seven organochlorine contaminants. DDT, banned for decades was one of the pesticide levels studied in relation to lower blood serum levels of vitamin D pre-hormone, 25 hydroxyvitamin D (25(OH)D), the standard by which vitamin D levels in the human body is assessed. Organochloride pesticides have been banned in the U.S. for decades, yet DDT has been found in countries where it has not been used.

Several Australian universities including the Menzies Research Institute together with the Norwegian Institute for Air Research (NILU) Tromso, Norway conducted a research study and found insufficiency in vitamin D across Australian populations is only partly explained by season and latitude. Vitamin D deficiencies were checked Winter/Spring in South-East Queensland, Geelong and Tasmania, with Tasmania showing the highest rate of Vitamin D deficiency at 67.3 per cent.

In Europe the latitudinal gradient goes the other way with lower prevalence of vitamin D insufficiency in northern Europe than southern Europe. Scandinavian countries are reputed to have very strict regulations in the use of pesticides and additives in food. Also, schoolchildren in Denmark have been weaned off processed food and these populations eat foods rich in vitamin D like dairy products and fish.

Vitamin D is metabolised by the liver and kidneys. It is converted into Calcidiol in the liver, part of which is converted into Calcitriol by the kidneys before Vitamin D can be used in our biochemistry. But an equally important job of the liver and kidneys is the expulsion of toxic chemicals from the body. Toxins accumulate in the liver to be transported in the blood to the kidneys for expulsion in the urine.

Naturally the intelligence in our bodies may choose saving our lives over absorbing vitamin D if there's an overload of toxins on our liver and kidneys. One in three Australians is supposed to be Vitamin D deficient. To make matters worse for us in Australia is our sulphur deficient soils as any agronomist can attest to (no volcanic activity here or near us for millions of years). Sulphur salts when active in our bodies, in their biochemical forms, ie. sodium sulphate, potassium sulphate and calcium sulphate work with other cleansing minerals in detoxification through our eliminative organs like the liver and kidneys. We are undersupplied in the very minerals which indirectly, in their cleansing action, may facilitate vitamin D absorption by freeing up the liver and kidneys from dealing with too many toxins.

Unfortunately since the passing of the Competition Reform Act 1995, by both major political parties,(I stood as a candidate for the Australian Democrats in 1996 and spoke on local radio about this bill, which the Democrats, Greens and Senator Brian Harradine voted against), our utilities have been privatised starting with Telecom into Telstra and it is not considered in the spirit of competition to stringently check the use of pesticides and other chemicals, particularly when used domestically and here in Tasmania by Forestry, unless there's a complaint. However, it is senseless to be concerned about escalating health costs and vitamin D insufficiency when we will not spend the money to mandatorily check foods as strictly as the Scandinavians are reputed to do.

Researching the articles for Tasmanian Life provided me with a timeline of information regarding mineral depletion in our foods and gave me a better understanding of what is happening to our health, particularly the young, whose requirements for growth and development is often not being met, compared with those of us born over 60 years ago. It was (1) the article "Plague of Plenty" in the November 2002 edition of the New Scientist that first alerted me, pointing out that soil scientists were finding trees leaving sizeable percentages of essential minerals in the soil and a further article pointing out that we are getting less than half the nutrients of previous generations. Then (2) in 2007, there was "Beneficial Effects of Potassium on Human Health" from the International Fertiliser Society pointing out that people today have only one third the potassium of previous generations. In April, 2012 (3) there was the ABC Catalyst program "Tree Deaths" where extremes of weather meant trees dying and then revived in West Australia by potassium phosphate and trace elements. Then (4) reading about further research by Arakli Loladze and other scientists, with food crops like rice and wheat leaving sizeable percentages of minerals in the soil and filling up with sugar when carbon dioxide is taken atmospherically.

~ Eleven ~

ARE WE CREATING NEW PROBLEMS?

We are living at a time of new names for conditions unheard of in previous generations.

Some months ago I read about Pyrrole disorder which shows up as a mauve colour on testing paper in urinalysis. It seems to be an undiagnosed feature of many behavioural and emotional disorders, including poor concentration, anxiety, mood swings, sensitivity to light and noise, stresses etc. etc.

When I read the list of symptoms I said to myself, but these are mostly potassium phosphate/magnesium phosphate symptoms. Children with this disorder seem to have problems absorbing zinc, magnesium and vitamin B6. Sometimes there are calcium phosphate and/or sodium phosphate or sodium sulphate symptoms too. Essentially it seems to be the lack of the minerals for growth, the phosphate minerals that provide also for the absorption of and interaction with vitamins and trace elements. If the macro minerals are inadequate, how can our bodies work with vitamins, enzyme systems etc. and the long complex processes that make hormones? I have observed how minerals over time seem to restore natural hormone function, even when defunct for years. Gut bacteria too, is being lauded today, but not the mineral compound responsible for ph balance and the right environment for healthy bacteria to thrive in.

Dr Maurice Blackmore taught that in treating chronic conditions, sodium phosphate or sodium sulphate is required to balance a prescribed formula. It is usually sodium phosphate which regulates the pH balance, which gets thrown out just as much by stress or grief as bad diet and symptoms for its need are so often present. How can we expect to grow healthy gut bacteria if we are acidic? It's all about balance and sodium phosphate is very much a balancing mineral compound. And we are not merely a being of separate organs and separate systems. Interaction and cooperation exist between all systems of the body. Health and balance seems to be life's purpose, or it is when adequately supported by the elements of life.

There is another name being bandied about for those not absorbing B vitamins, demonstrating to me and other mineral prescribers, the unravelling of our metabolisms, yet we bypass the most basic biochemical processes. We do not know better than Nature, which has created us. We should check minerals like magnesium, and with children, calcium with sodium phosphate as well, before we decide about leaky gut or malabsorption for vitamin B and/or trace elements. Once the basic mineral balance is right, better absorption of vitamins and trace elements more easily occurs.

Basic biochemistry, being the foundation for everything in life, therefore should be the first line of treatment. I've never known it to fail, unless I make a mistake in the prescription, or try to force the pace. And I've learned never to forget that with a severely debilitated person, one must prescribe minimally at first, to lay the foundation for them to later benefit with higher doses - one avoids flogging a dead horse. If very occasionally the patient is taking the minerals at the prescribed doses and not responding, I have made a mistake. The minerals are always needed, but I must have got the balance wrong for that person.

Back in the 1970s in Melbourne a woman came to the clinic, who had been in a concentration camp during the second world war. She had never resolved her digestive problems. She was perhaps the only person at that time who did not respond on Blackmores celloids. I've not forgotten her and wonder if she may have responded on the tissue salts, the homeopathic minerals, 6x dose, which were originally used by Dr. William Schussler, who used the homeopathic dose to infiltrate the cell to encourage absorption where the mineral supplies in the cell had become too eroded to properly attract the minerals to them. Perhaps using the 6x homeopathic dose until better absorption was achieved, might have been followed by the celloids and finally attaining a good digestive system.

Maurice Blackmore decided that minerals were required in a pharmacological dose. He reasoned that because Europe has dolomite and limestone rich soils being so much younger geologically than Australia, the homeopathic dose in Europe may work there, but Blackmores Laboratories used the homeopathic mix with the pharmacological dose for Australia. Les Fisher included the 6x homeopathic formula with the pharmacological dose for his tablets, which are ratified with the Therapeutic Goods Authority and I use both products.

Dr William Schussler and the doctors who worked with him, had found that the minerals cannot be destroyed, even in combustion, so when death occurs, the minerals in the being that once lived are taken back by nature for further life purposes. WE CANNOT CREATE NOR DESTROY THE MINERAL ELEMENTS OF LIFE that are major activators of our body processes. All else can combust or rot away, but not the mineral elements. This understanding should be enough for us to put the macro minerals first, particularly when our children are developing debilitating problems, which were hardly seen in my generation.

For nearly 50 years now I have seen how the mineral elements regenerate life and continue to do so over the decades, sometimes even with people severely depleted in the first place.

For myself therefore, this "new" pyrrole disorder is a symptom of macro mineral depletion, particularly phosphate directed minerals, the building blocks of potassium, magnesium, calcium, sodium, iron. Correctly prescribed for the specific symptoms only, the emotional and behavioural symptoms respond quickly. Because our foods and soils provide less than half the essential elements than previously, these days, people may do better with a maintenance dose, once health is attained, or topping up with minerals, particularly after growth spurts with children.

Over recent years, a psychologist has sent a number of children and adolescents to me for help with their physical health. I wonder if many of them may have tested positively for pyrrole because of so many of their symptoms. But why do the test when decades of experience points to balance once specific mineral compounds are working.

It was a bit horrifying to meet young teenagers who could sleep for 14 hours and still wake tired. There were often many potassium phosphate/magnesium phosphate symptoms apart from allergy, digestive or circulation problems also often present.

One of these girls I remember well because the first thing I wrote down was that she could not stop crying. She also got Raynaud's phenomenon and the skin on her feet split and froze in winter. I saw her first in June (our first month of winter), then 3 weeks later. She had become happier, sleeping better and her circulation was improved. Again I saw her in another 3 weeks, the day before she was due to do an exam. She came with her grandmother and she had a smile on her face. Her grandmother said she had not seen this girl so happy for a long time. She was looking forward to her exam, no tears since the first couple of weeks and no Raynaud's and it was the end of July (usually our coldest month). I realised that the girl was so unhappy because she had found it so difficult to do well at school. It took only 2 mineral compounds, four times daily to bring things into balance for her.

Another girl felt depressed because she thought she was failing at high school, particularly in Maths and Science. Fourteen hours of sleep was not enough to cure her fatigue. She over-ate (indiscriminate eating requires potassium phosphate : sweet things in particular require magnesium phosphate), yet always had an empty feeling no matter how much food she consumed. Over the next few months her other symptoms improved. She was going to a well known girls' school. In an exam at school, her results were so good that her teacher said "What are you doing? You are even good now in subjects you have not previously done well in". So the girl explained about the minerals (3 different compounds in her case) and how all her symptoms had almost gone. The teacher asked the rest of the class if any of them had any of these symptoms and over half the class put up their hands.

When this young girl told me the story, I thought back to the teacher who asked "How can you teach children with a 5 minute attention span?" Here in Southern Tasmania, the population is largely descended from British and Aborigine inhabitants. After generations living on this soil, where there's no iodine and little of essential macro minerals and trace elements apart from iron, I am wondering about increasing learning difficulties in our children. These days the Aborigine population lives mostly on much the same food as us (forgetting their kelp inheritance : such a shame when they were such a beautiful well-muscled race of people). On the Mainland, about half the population are new Australians, many of whom seem to be doing quite well educationally. I wonder how many generations of being undernourished with macro minerals it takes for epigenetic pathways to become less effective in gene expression!

I advise people to include sea vegetables in their diet and their gardens, for iodine and all the trace elements. For university students when studying, I remember Adelle Davis and the value of brewers yeast in unsweetened pineapple juice with its valuable digestive enzymes. Often students study for 50 minutes, then 10 minutes break and the brewers yeast in pineapple juice in the break time clears the brain they say, making them ready for more study. As well as the B vitamins, there is protein, potassium and other trace elements in the brewers yeast that comes from hops used to make beer.

We used to go to the brewery to buy malt cones (also full of B vitamins) for the horses. So we took care of our horses, but what about our children? Rarely are children today given cod liver oil to help the immune system and calcium absorption : no more sulphur and treacle and here in Tasmania, no more iodine drops for children. They are thought to get enough iodine from what's added to salt.

But when there are deficits of other nutrients, particularly minerals, the body's ability to absorb seems to diminish, even for people who learn and take particular care to eat only an exemplary diet. These people usually respond quickly and sometimes come to experience a level of health not previously enjoyed. Most of us today consider it normal to simply live with irritating symptoms, or take a pill to help ignore it. Fewer people today are bursting with joie de vivre. Too many are depressed and sometimes suicidal, displaying deterioration in mental as well as physical health.

Current treatments for pyrrole remind me of modern medicine which has become often very good at the quick fix, but addressing the obvious without going deeper. When one forgets about the name attached and delves into a history of the individual symptoms, one can discover a progression that will lead back to the basics - the minerals. As I have said to my patients over the years, "the symptoms are there for a purpose, like pain." They can be suppressed which can put more stress on the body. Of course suppression can also allow the body a rest from pain, which if it is able, may eventually lead to healing. But I have come to believe in the real value of the symptoms to arrive at the basic elements for life and more complete healing and re-generation with the required minerals.

~ Twelve ~

SKIN THE OUTER ORGAN MAY TAKE TIME.

I recently heard on ABC Radio National, a story about Sir Winston Churchlll who got pneumonia rather badly during the second world war. He refused the new drugs and insisted on being treated with the Sulphonamides. As we know, he recovered. Sulphonamides apparently are not used much these days because they are believed to cause skin problems.

Sulphonamides are synthetic sulphur minerals. In treating many skin conditions like psoriasis, sulphur minerals are invaluable, (not synthetic), but in the natural format, the cation/anion relationship. Potassium sulphate is most often required to heal up psoriasis, particularly in hot, sweaty people. Some skin conditions of course are lymphatic and need both the sulphur salts and potassium chloride and sometimes sulphur salts are nor called for.

I thought about my brother who was a skinny little kid and he got boils that were so deep, they went through to the bone. He went regularly to the Brisbane General Hospital for penicillin injections into his bottom, the only place there was any flesh to inject into. A year went by and there was no improvement.

One day someone said to my mother "Give him a teaspoon of molasses each day". To our great surprise, there was one more small boil and then no more. After this my father made two jugs of drink each work and school morning. One had a big tablespoon of molasses mixed into boiled water. The one to follow was citrus juice and honey mixed with hot water. I thought it diabolical that we had to have these drinks before breakfast each morning. No one else did. I should say that my mother was very concerned about good health and she bought our bread from the Sanitarium Health Shop in Brisbane, the only health shop at that time and we had nuts, dried fruits and lots of fresh fruits too. The only time I was happy about our wholemeal bread was on Mondays, when at school our bread was still edible while the white bread sandwiches of our friends was stale and hard (no preservatives then but I am sure we were healthier without the preservatives). My brother developed great stamina and scored 5 and 6 tries in Rugby League in Junior and Senior League. I can't remember which score was for which League. We all had good skin and I had no trouble with my skin in puberty, which was commented on for its clarity. The sulphur minerals in molasses today are sometimes taken out. I can't understand this when Australian soils are often so lacking in sulphur salts. We certainly need them to help purification in our liver and kidneys and surely it's much better to get natural sulphur salts than the synthetic sulphur salts in sulphonamides.

A young man who worked at the university came to see me not long ago. He had had aggravating red bumps on his skin for nearly 2 decades and skin specialists had not helped. But he said it was because of how I had helped his mother that he came to me. I was not a practitioner he would choose to go to. His mother was taking the minerals for her cervicals. She had been due for surgery and her condition had improved so much, that her surgeon said to see how she goes and to come back if she needed the surgery, which had not happened. This young man was not easy to get symptoms from. When I asked him about his circulation, he said it was good. Later in discussion, I learned that when he went diving in a wet suit with friends, he was first out of the water. I gave him two compounds, one for the lymphatic system and pH balance and the other for the circulation. When he returned in 3 weeks, he said he had taken the 2 compounds to the skin specialist the previous week and demanded to know why they had not been prescribed by the skin specialist. His skin was clear for the first time in many years. He refused to believe me that the specialist may not know about this basic biochemistry.

Year 12 and university students can sometimes have quite nasty psoriasis contributed to by lack of sleep, poor diet and stress. One asks the questions to find how the individual can be helped. I remember one university student whose face had been swollen for some time with big blackheads, displaying a lymphatic problem as well as the need for purifying sulphur minerals. If stress is contributing to the condition, that must also be addressed. I rang this girl a few weeks after her first lot of minerals. She said she was disappointed. She had got another round of big pimples. I asked her what the skin itself was like. Could she tell if anything else was developing. She said the skin seemed smoother and then felt happier because nothing more seemed to be coming out. I explained that the skin is an eliminative organ and one must allow the skin to push out whatever is there while creating with the minerals an environment that doesn't produce the skin problem in the first place. We talked about her food and sleep.

She was already sleeping better since taking the minerals. She stayed on the minerals a few months longer, just to be sure she really had got rid of the psoriasis.

It's a good experience for students to learn how to help themselves, that one can do a great deal to help oneself. This is also apparent for those who develop bronchial troubles in the winter. People love to find they do not have to be a victim to things.

Years earlier at Edwards Pharmacy I had treated a woman for many symptoms she had not recovered from following radio and chemotherapy for cancer. She was aggravated that she had to wear a wig. She lost her hair following the cancer treatment. Over months, on the minerals, her health improved well. Within a year her eyebrows grew back. I had told her that we can grow a second head of hair, even if the original roots were destroyed (happened to me as a child from radium therapy to my scalp and I became bald for months). She was much encouraged by the return of her eyebrows but it took a few months longer for the hair follicles to reappear on her scalp. Then she grew a thick head of lovely, wavy hair and wrote to the skin specialist to tell him not to tell people they could not grow another head of hair.

Skin problems can be frustrating to treat, particularly bad eczema in children and I have seen a few who've taken minerals on and off for years until puberty, when finally beautiful skin has arrived. It seems to me that the skin, as the outer organ gets the benefit of the minerals after internal needs are satisfied.

My memoir follows the principles of Narrative therapy, a valuable tool in Psychology where one can learn from the narrative of experiences that hopefully the reader may relate to. This is not a textbook, even though I often write about minerals prescribed in particular instances. I hope above all that these stories will be taken seriously, and those interested will find mineral therapists or information in textbooks or on the internet. Psychology has shown that the psychologist as sounding board is invaluable, and likewise we may not alone, without the help of another valued person and opinion, accurately assess our own needs.

With an escalating health budget, surely the time has come to check and support our soils, foods and basic biochemistry. One day hopefully, basic biochemistry will be used to support all other methods of medicine and we'll not only legislate but actively enforce environmental protection we pay lip service to today.

~ Thirteen ~

A PHILOSOPHY ABOUT THE ELEMENTS OF LIFE.

THE TRUTH IS INCONTROVERTIBLE. MALICE MAY ATTACK IT. IGNORANCE MAY DERIDE IT, BUT IN THE END, THERE IT IS. -
WINSTON CHURCHILL.
(PERMISSION NOT SOUGHT)

David Attenborough has entertained and educated us with so many wonderful programs about our world. There is one that particularly resonates with me about the Serengeti National Park. Mount Kilimanjaro with its three volcanic cones fertilises the Serengeti Plain from these volcanos and it is the chosen birth place for African animals for miles around. They come in peace with each other for the birth of their offspring to benefit from the mineral rich vegetation. How can it be that with the development of artificial and synthetic medicine, we do not have the instinctual knowledge and intelligence of these other species!! How many of us ensure best health which should precede our pregnancies, to ensure a good foundation for the next generation? Or are we indeed The Unconscious Civilisation, so called by John Rawlston Saul?

Australians were once known as one of the world's healthiest people. Our Aborigines were usually not included in our medical statistics, but we white people were often only a few generations away from European ancestors, who came from mineral rich soils and unprocessed foods. Yet our grandparents knew about lack of sulphur in Australian soils that were far removed from proximity to volcanic activity and it was quite usual to regularly give children sulphur and treacle or molasses. These simple intelligent precautions are today largely ignored along with cod liver oil for good bone growth. Instead our health has slipped drastically according to world statistics and we have increasing liver and kidney disease and now the highest rate of allergies in the world. Sulphur acts as an anion directing the actions of cations of potassium, calcium and sodium for specific cleansing and healing purposes. But basic biochemistry is also largely ignored. I heard James Lovelock on a radio program describe Australia's soils as "ancient and friable" that would not stand up to climate change, which our farmers are now discovering. How therefore can we expect to be healthy when we ignore what may be essentially lacking and don't understand how climate change is interfering with how nutrients are absorbed by plants? If koalas are threatened, not only by loss of habitat, but diminishing of water and minerals in the gum leaves they eat, then what is happening to the rest of us?

ABC Four Corners program "Swallowing It" (13/2/2017) started off saying that Australians are spending billions on unproven vitamins and supplements. Apparently Australians are spending more on vitamins and supplements than on drugs. People are not stupid. Neither are we so unconscious as sometimes seems to be the case. We are forced to spend twice, supporting a medical system which we find unsustaining without the help of extra money spent on products we find beneficial. Why is the medical bureaucracy not questioning what might be done to benefit our health naturally? Do we really know better than Nature? Education is key. There are doctors who do their own research into natural medicine, just like many members of the public. Producers of vitamins and supplements do not deserve criticism from those who accept products from spurious trials. It's dishonest to remove people from the first trial of a new drug, who have reacted badly and then use those who remain in the following trials to accredit a new product, which is then supposed to be medically validated.

Despite what is ignored, in fact what is most powerful of all is an underlying philosophy to the Elements of Life which unites all living beings, through macro minerals and trace elements. This is a wonderful philosophy because it demonstrates the power of the life force which is perhaps best understood by science through James Lovelock's Gaia philosophy, how Gaia has maintained for 3.6 billion years, a balance in our atmosphere, (including lower CO_2 levels than now) - a protection of life's environment, often foolishly taken for granted. Isn't climate swinging between extremes of hot and cold, a demonstration of Nature trying to cope with imbalances caused by rising temperatures and CO_2? The minerals too work in conjunction with each other, utilising vitamins and other nutrients, and also aim for stability and optimum health of living creatures, just like our environment which has protected and maintained the systems of life for such a long time.

Some ancient religions like Buddhism respect all living matter, but the significance of the minerals, in their perpetuation of human life was best described as Biochemistry by its founders who were Christians, those elements essential for our lives which we have taken for granted. With drug medicines, we can disguise from ourselves painful learning experiences. Bob Hawke, a past prime minister of ours, famously used the word "wanker" about someone. Well haven't we become a species of wankers, when we can disguise from ourselves, unpleasant realities of life and behave as if our abused environment is maintaining life as it once did? In many cultures the future for the next generation took precedence over the instant personal gratification of today. How many of us are like the frog in a pot of water coming to the boil, not consciously registering what's happening?

Mineral therapy is based on a philosophy of hope and faith in life. Unfortunately much of modern medicine is based on a philosophy of fear. "We must fight nature". This is a battle we can never win. Some of science is working with nature. Heavy metals are being considered to cleanse the Derwent River, Tasmania using a form of sulphur salts. What a pity it is not understood that sodium sulphate in small regular doses may expel heavy metals from the human body and helps the health of our liver and kidneys, particularly now that we know that liver disease, like many others is escalating. Potassium chloride is used in heart by-pass surgery and I've heard of potassium recently used in hospitals for leukaemia. But minerals are required to MAINTAIN our daily health in small, regular amounts like our bodies are designed to absorb from food. We remain unconscious of the fact that we are more and more suffering from "hidden hunger" as there are less and less of these elements available to us.

We don't want to believe in God. Yet it is obvious to anyone working with the elements of life, that there is an over-riding intelligence directing how these elements work, their priorities in healing and their ability to provide balance when it has been upset by our actions or other forces. This intelligence always tries for equilibrium, as James Lovelock found in his atmospheric research. (He was the scientist who made the instrument with which we measured the hole in the ozone). To me it is all about the life force and its power.

Nearly 10 years ago I flew back from England with a young German scientist. She said she was working at an American university and was about to visit a university in Melbourne with her research. She was working with oncology drugs. I told her that it concerned me that drugs pass through our bodies into the rivers and oceans poisoning the environment. She said her research showed that certain oncology drugs can work just as effectively in much smaller doses which would greatly minimise what escapes into the environment. That sounded wonderful to me, but has anyone heard anything about this research being adopted by the drug companies?

Nearly 50 years has demonstrated to me, how a small number of minerals have both immediate affects on acute symptoms with 2 hourly doses and long term 2 or 3 times daily doses for thousands of people with chronic problems, rebuilding their health. It may once have seemed too good to be true. But the truth is simple. These elements I believe, are the spearhead of epigenetic processes. Working in pharmacies, I found myself delving into every health product to find the mineral or minerals which might promote normal epigenetic activation. Methylation is an epigenetic mechanism used by our cells to control gene expression and methylation starts with minerals like sulphur.

I am not attracted to scientific reductionism which mineral therapy may appear to be, when we use a few of only eleven mineral compounds as a basis for healing and interaction with other chemical reactions in the body, prescribed strictly for specific symptoms. Yet our very complexity is predicated on the most basic elements, which to me means it's better to come back to the basics which will support any other modality of healing while allowing Nature to do her work. The human body works just like the planet. What is altered in one organ will mean reorganisation elsewhere in the body. Builders certainly understand that the foundations are critical when building a house.

But what worries me most and has become the driving force of this book is, global warming and atmospheric carbon dioxide and seemingly, the effect on our food plants. Associate Professor, Mathematical Biologist & Quantitive Ecologist, Arakli Loladze and other scientists have studied the percentages of minerals left behind in the soil because plants seem to prefer CO_2, and crops like wheat, rice and hundreds of other food and wild plants have been found to be filling up with sugar instead of minerals. And we are worried about obesity and diabetes!! This increase in atmospheric CO_2 goes back to the industrial revolution but there's little awareness of an increasing effect on plants, apart from in plant sciences. Or are the changes directly occurring because of global warming? Increasing temperatures may mean increasing CO_2, and minerals like potassium, as botanists well know are decreasingly absorbed when soils are too wet or too dry. Maybe plants more easily absorb CO_2 from the atmosphere than various essential minerals from the soil, as rising temperatures cause more extreme weather conditions and soils too become more extreme between wet and dry.

One of my greatest concerns is how mineral depletion goes hand in hand with acceptance and adjustment to lower levels of health., physical, emotional and intellectual. When potassium phosphate is lacking, a person may experience lack of incentive, courage and stamina to face life's tribulations. Anxiety and depression also become increasingly present. We have created a great mess through greed and inattention to results of our exploitation of the planet. We have sinkholes, actually joining together in West Texas, terrible ocean pollution etc. and know we can no longer put off dealing with these excesses which we can put a stop to, but Nature herself will ultimately restore order, with or without us. If we become heavy handed, we may cause more destruction in a system of complexity we do not properly understand. We can probably store CO_2 so far, but like storing radioactive waste, this is not a real answer, when temperatures that are continuing to increase mean climatic excesses leading to structural instability of land as well as sea.

My other great concern is the world's population excess. NASA has stated that we are overusing Earth's resources, so birth control becomes essential. Thom Hartmann in "The Last Hours of Ancient Sunlight" points out that our hunter gatherer ancestors knew which plants to use for contraception so did not overpopulate the land they needed to sustain them. I had heard this from a retired pioneer missionary in New Guinea. She always regretted that she could not find out about the plant the native women used for birth control and now they may have lost the knowledge. Condoning out of control greed seems to have turned us into a breed of mindless, meddling monkeys who worship an aberrant, selfish intellect. Fortunately there are many of us who do our best to face the reality created around us and who love life enough to unceasingly work for restoration and understanding and real value of the laws of Nature. As my memoir shows, Nature is powerfully regenerative.

We must wonder when the tipping point will come, when it will be a waste of time to add nutrients we know depleted soils need if the plants are leaving more and more in the soil. My great concern is that in losing essential minerals, we can expect our mental and physical abilities to decline and we may become less capable of dealing with the increasing destruction to life. Surely drastically reducing CO_2 is the first priority. We did something about the hole in the ozone. But even a drastic reduction in CO_2 will still leave life at a deficit for some time while Nature attempts to clean up.

Like many others I wonder if many of us have learned how to think. My mother's brothers were all teachers. The one who became a politician asked me a question once when I was about twelve. I started to answer "Mum thinks ....". "Never mind what your mother thinks. What do you think?" I was irritated at the time. Thinking things through for oneself may be difficult and as we learn and experience more, our thinking may change. But at least we are not abnegating what we think to others, particularly our elites, whose concerns may not be ours. I imagined that at university one would be encouraged to think and question. University was at the beginning of economic change in the early 1990s when I was there. Now students are often taught by graduating students with many university professors encouraged to take a redundancy. It has become a degree mill and you had better answer their exams with exactly what you have been taught, not waste the time of the overworked examiners with too much additional stuff if you want good marks. Universities in Australia today seem to no longer encourage thinking and questioning.

I particularly wonder about what to me are very pertinent questions about epidemics. The world flu epidemic in 1917 came towards the end of the first world war with so much disruption. But more than this was the wholesale introduction of chemicals like mustard gas and so much destruction not only to people, but to animals, plants etc., diminished fresh food to millions. We know how volcanic eruptions and earthquakes affect life on this planet and so does war. That flu epidemic is sometimes spoken of but not questions about the underlying factors. What about the polio epidemic between the world wars and in the 1950s. The wholesale introduction of coca cola (sugar in amounts not previously experienced) is rarely questioned as a contributing factor to the polio epidemic. And what about staphylococcos in hospitals? Operating theatres once had walls, ceilings, everything washed between surgeries. Florence Nightingale revolutionised hospitals by teaching extreme cleanliness. In an overcrowded world, extreme cleanliness is more necessary than ever and so is clean air. Our health is dependant on the food we eat, the water we drink and the air we breathe. We know that our soils are overworked and depleted, yet we are foolish enough to take for granted that our foods contain the elements of life we need, despite our awareness of so many environmental changes for the worse.

People power here in Australia has prevailed to force politicians and our banks to face up to cheating the public. As more and more people and organisations understand our sins against Nature and how the health and stamina of ourselves and all life is being destroyed, people power as always, can provide the impetus for change. We can start with banning coal, our biggest producer of CO_2.

About 3 years ago NASA space scientists researched how we are using Earth's resources and predicted that our civilisation will collapse within 30 years (30 years of civilisation left NASA). They stated that it would be our elites as in ancient Rome and the Mayan civilisation, who will be most responsible for this collapse, those who avoid the struggles so many people have, cocooning themselves in luxury. The same argument applies to the loss of essential nutrients which those who can afford to will take in tablet form, avoiding the reality of collapse of nutrients in plants and animals.

I hope this memoir is not tilting at windmills. But perhaps it may contribute to action and understanding about life's dependence on the elements of life. When I was about 9 years old, our teacher who was an Englishman called Mr Cooper, said to me "Irene, stop tilting at windmills like Don Quixote." I don't know what I had said, and didn't understand what he meant. Am I once again tilting at windmills? I am 78 years old now and have felt more and more driven to write this memoir. The life force is so powerful with a huge capacity for regeneration. My faith in life and its capacities for regeneration is my wish for our children and grandchildren, now and a future where all life in our animals, plants and environment is loved and cared for, appreciated for its gift to us.

EXAMPLE OF MINERAL HEALTH MIRACLE

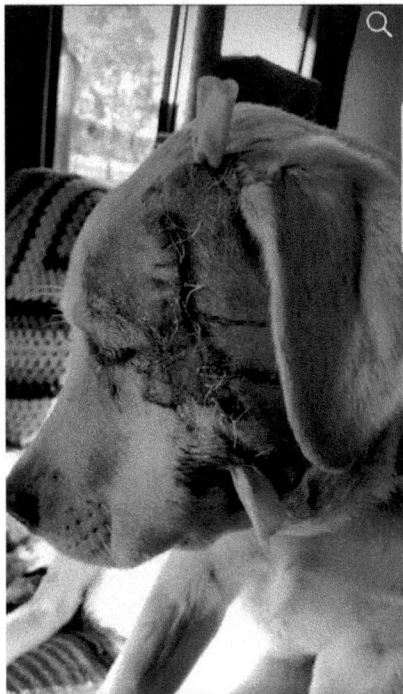

Spencer after 2 operations and taken off antibiotics because of his age

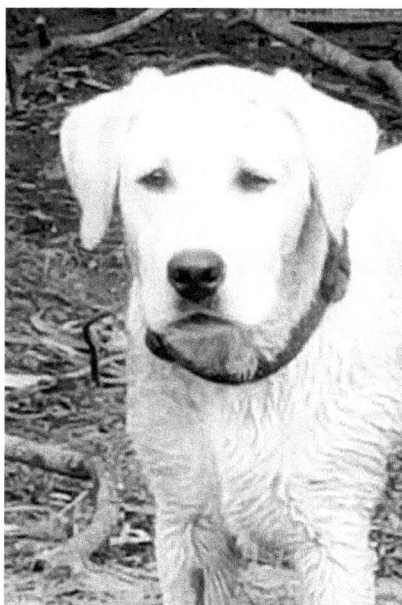

Spencer today after one 84 tablet container of mineral tablets with the potassium and sulphur cleansing mineral salts in biochemical format

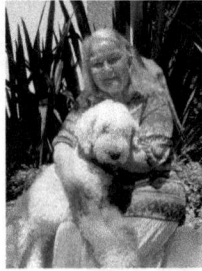

ABOUT THE AUTHOR

Irene lives in a retirement village overlooking Hobart's Rivulet. She still sees a few past and new patients, but today there a number of mineral therapists in Hobart, and readily available over the counter quality mineral formulas. Today Irene is working for acknowledgment politically, for laws to forbid production of toxins destructive to life and not biodegradable.

Global warming leads to Hidden Hunger as extremes of rain and drought mean less and less mineral absorption by plants, the main food source for all of life. She hopes her memoir helps to consolidate action, particularly from Medicine, perhaps the last scientific body that believes we can succeed against Nature.